Adolescents with Language and Literacy Needs: A Shoulder-to-Shoulder Collaboration

Adolescents with Language and Learning Needs: A Shoulder-to-Shoulder Collaboration

Sandra Tattershall, Ph.D.
Language and Learning Center
Florence, Kentucky

SINGULAR

TM

THOMSON LEARNING

Australia Canada Mexico Singapore Spain United Kingdom United States

SINGULAR

———✳———™

THOMSON LEARNING

Adolescents with Language and Learning Needs: A Shoulder-to-Shoulder Collaboration
by
Sandra Tattershall, Ph.D.

Health Care Publishing Director:
William Brottmiller

Channel Manager:
Jennifer McAvey

Executive Editor:
Cathy L. Esperti

Production Editor:
Mary Colleen Liburdi

Acquisitions Editor:
Candice Janco

Illustrator:
Dick Hataway

Editorial Assistant:
Maria D'Angelico

Executive Marketing Manager:
Dawn F. Gerrain

Library of Congress
Cataloging-in-Publication Data
On File

ISBN 1-5659-3888-7

NOTICE TO THE READER

Contents

Foreword

Sandra Tattershall's book is the tenth in the school-age children series. Like others in the series, it embodies the themes I envisioned when first asked to serve as series editor more than a decade ago—collaboration, contextually based intervention, change, and relevance. Tattershall's unique voice resonates through the printed word. Both her sense of humor and practical good sense can be found here.

Anyone who has heard Sandra Tattershall speak knows her special mix of caring and respect for adolescents who are struggling with the demands of school. In this book, Tattershall describes her methods for working with adolescents in a "shoulder-to-shoulder" problem-solving approach. The book is intended for an audience that includes students, parents, and general education teachers, as well as speech-language pathologists and other special service providers. In Tattershall's approach, adolescents are primary collaborative partners in addressing their own social interaction and academic challenges. Chapter 4, in fact, was written with adolescents (among others) in mind as the intended audience. It presents a series of case descriptions that students can read and discuss to understand their own situations and to reduce their feelings of aloneness and difference.

In this book, Tattershall also describes how to work with adolescents in a manner that is contextually based and relevant to their everyday learning needs. She helps students, and those who work with them, grasp the importance of communication issues in language processing and academic learning. She presents methods and strategies for understanding classroom discourse and knowing what to do with the language of homework.

In the first three chapters, Tattershall shows how to connect language processing goals to real world knowledge and specific academic goals. She presents the approach as individualized and modifiable for individual students. In Chapters 7 and 8, she describes learning principles designed to help students become aware of what they do in real life learning as a basis for improving their language processing in academic learning. Throughout the book, Tattershall expands on these issues and tells how to apply language and communication intervention strategies to improve students' functioning in the important contexts of their lives. One of my favorite features is her sharing of her own clinical discourse—the words she uses to help adolescents see themselves in a new light and to advance their use of language skills and strategies.

The underlying theme of change is also represented throughout the book. Tattershall expects that intervention can yield differences in students' lives and that these differences can enhance their potential for further change and development. In Chapters 5 and 6, Tattershall focuses on the use of diagnostic tools in the decision making and goal setting process. She emphasizes the importance of all collaborative partners, including students and their parents, in understanding the implications of findings of the formal assessment process and how to augment it with informal assessment data to guide the process of change.

The outcome of Tattershall's approach to information sharing is a highly practical, readable, and relevant book, with information and suggestions for working with adolescents in a way that will yield meaningful changes in their lives. I recommend it highly as a resource for anyone concerned about meeting the needs of adolescents with communication and learning issues. It is a particular honor to have the work of a respected colleague and valued friend as one of the culminating volumes in the school-age children series. I appreciate Tattershall's dedication to bringing the book to life, and I admire her ability to do it so well.

Nickola Wolf Nelson
Series Editor

Preface

Working with adolescents and young adults has been an education for me as a professional. I don't recall learning much about this age group in my formal classwork but I have been fortunate in meeting a variety of youngsters who have been my "teachers" since then.

Because they are struggling with communication and learning, the adolescents I see can be more fragile, defensive, defeated, or guarded than their more fortunate peers. In spite of their difficulties, however, these youngsters have provided insights that seem applicable to many students but are unavailable elsewhere. I hope to share many of these insights in this book.

I have written this book for those who work with adolescents and young adults—for speech-language pathologists (SLPs), educators of those with special needs, regular classroom teachers, those who work in counseling, those who guide adolescents in transitions to college and work, and for parents who are working hard to understand and help their children.

Readers will be provided with an effective approach for working with adolescents having difficulty in understanding and producing extended discourse. The shoulder-to-shoulder relationship inherent in this approach defines the adult and adolescent roles necessary for effective collaboration. Each person, in this approach, contributes to a joint effort using the specific strategies presented for improving language and learning in academic, vocational, and social settings. Problem solving is the focus of the work, clarifying for adolescents how to work on current difficulties and guiding practice in skills for lifelong learning. In the attempts to identify and solve problems, the necessary communication between adolescents and their adult partners results in effective language learning and practice with extended discourse.

Chapters 1 through 3 describe the shoulder-to-shoulder stance, the problem solving focus, the importance of connecting real world knowledge and skills to academics and adolescent's need for learning specific language processing strategies for extended discourse. Reading and discussing the first three chapters will introduce and help define the shoulder-to-shoulder problem solving approach which is to be adjusted and personalized for particular adolescents and situations.

In Chapter 4, descriptions of a variety of clients will provoke questions and many "aha's" as adolescents recognize themselves through others' experience. This chapter will help dispel the lonely feeling so common to those who feel different and distanced from others. As students, professionals, and parents read about other adolescents' difficulties, lists of similar problems for the student in question can be generated.

Chapters 5 and 6 should be helpful for professionals and parents who are trying to evaluate and select diagnostic tools. The information in these chapters clarifies how these tools can guide the problem solving process. Adolescents also need to understand what is being done to and for them in the diagnostic stage; these chapters can help. Many adolescents will, of course, be more interested in the results than the process of diagnostics. Parents and adolescents can appreciate in reading this part of the book how their observations contribute to the diagnostic findings and make standardized scores more meaningful. Parents sometimes seem confused by test results and may need to learn about what is being done, why and how final suggested plans relate to the findings. Parents, professionals and adolescents may have a better understanding of the specifics of a diagnostic report, such as its recommendations or final plan, if they have an opportunity to read about the process in these sections. Adolescents need to be reminded in discussions that even though diagnostic tools are important in the beginning of a collaboration, the problem solving process will be ongoing and plans may change with new observations.

Chapters 7 and 8 direct the planning in problem solving with adolescents. The Learning Principles can be invaluable in enhancing adolescents' awareness of what they do in real life learning and can serve as a base for improving their language processing in academic learning. Communicating with adolescents can be facilitated with these principles guiding observations and discussion. For instance, it is rewarding to see adolescents appreciate that they regularly apply the "What-So What" principle in their interactions with others. They rarely let a notable or confusing statement (the "What") go unchallenged in conversation without trying to understand it ("So what"). Because they typically go beyond the statement to understand the reasons behind the comment, adolescents usually remember what is said in conversation. This example and others from typical daily communication allow adult collaborators to promote the need to question and understand the reasons underlying academic concepts. The Learning Principles provide continuing referents for adolescents who are trying to effectively process the extended discourse of school.

Chapter 8 provides the real "meat" for working on extended discourse with adolescents who have been struggling in school without knowing what to do. Those youngsters who have stared at their homework without understanding or have applied what seems to be a universal study strategy—"Go over it"—will learn better, more specific strategies. Of course, students will not learn these strategies by simply reading about or listening to explanations. Most of the adolescents we know have been "told" many things that have not worked for them in school. They need both to be shown how and guided in practicing the strategies in this chapter using easy materials first to allow focus on new ways to process. When they show appreciation for how and why to apply a strategy, they will need guided practice in using the same strategy with more challenging materials and tasks from their current curriculum. They will need observation and discussion to ensure that they truly understand a strategy and/or to allow for the necessary fine tuning or modification in light of their learning styles and demands of particular tasks. This chapter provides a review of strategies that have been taught and practiced first—a check of understanding beyond the quick "I've got it" response so typical of some adolescents I have known. In so many cases, adolescents with limited natural talent in language processing have been included in fast moving classroom activities without checking their understanding. No one, including the students themselves, can be sure of what has been learned. After discovery and learning of strategies followed by practice, students may need to read the descriptions of these strategies. They should then be able to explain their understanding of these strategies for extended discourse. Reading about the strategies may clarify misconceptions and explaining in their own words should aid the storing of new information. The "Tutor–Tutee" learning principle (becoming the Tutor by explaining) can be applied using Chapter 8 for review.

Chapter 9 should help professionals appreciate the efficacy of using this shoulder-to-shoulder problem solving approach with a variety of populations in the specific teaching and guided practice of strategies for processing extended discourse—the language that has often been unavailable to at risk adolescents and has stopped their progress in learning.

Chapter 10 guides adolescents, their parents, and professionals in devising appropriate accommodations for work and school transitions. This section should help adolescents and young adults who have gained an understanding of their own needs through the shoulder-to-shoulder problem solving collaboration to know what accommodations are necessary and how to advocate for themselves in school and at work. The success of the collaboration between professionals and adolescents with special needs requires that everyone understand what is needed and how to ensure that these accommodations are in place and to appreciate that monitoring and adjusting plans are essential, that problem solving is an ongoing process in life, in school and on the job.

When Nikki Nelson invited me to write this book, she urged me to include, whenever possible, quotes to show how I communicate with my adolescent clients. I hope those who read and use this book can hear my way of communicating with adolescents coming through my writing. More importantly, I hope that the voices and specific insights of my adolescent and young adult clients can be heard. Even though they have come with limited language, they have been eloquent in contributing to my understanding of what they need and what works in helping them. I hope the readers of this book also profit from these insights.

Prologue

Brent was conscientious about his homework. He always did it and he always handed it in on time. He also had an excellent memory and, as a junior in high school, stored many pieces of information. He could provide answers for questions requiring isolated facts or trivia but not for those requiring in-depth understanding or application of information. He memorized because he was good at it; because that was what he thought he was supposed to do; and because memorizing was the only study strategy he knew. Unfortunately, this approach to learning had its limitations for Brent. Although he worked hard to collect and store information, what he learned was always out of context and of little use to him at test time. He was resentful, that in spite of completing his daily work and studying hard, he was not doing well in school. Brent needed help.

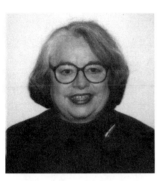

About the Author

Sandra S. Tattershall, Ph.D./CCC is director of the Language & Learning Center, a private practice. Her work sites have included working at the Children's Hospital School for Aphasic Children in Washington, D.C., in Fairfax County Public Schools, at the Louisville Deaf-Oral Preschool, and at the Cincinnati Speech and Hearing Center. She completed a clinical year at the Cincinnati Center for Developmental Disabilities, an interdisciplinary diagnostic center. Dr. Tattershall has been interested for many years in the language processing inherent in learning. She began collaborating with teachers in the early 80's to find ways to facilitate language processing within classroom scripts and within written language. She is now collaborating directly with children to enhance their awareness of their own processing and to expand their use of language strategies for school. She has presented frequently on the topic of academic language and continues to add to her own understanding.

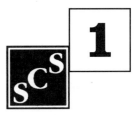

Working with Adolescents: An Overview

There is a comedian, I am told, who promises to review in twenty minutes, all the information those in his audience will remember ten years after high school graduation. Although this provocative statement is intended to get a laugh, the implication is serious—we don't retain much academic content from school.

The cultural literacy movement has posed a variation on this point, that is, that students often do not learn information in the first place, the kind of information that literate folks should know " ... the basic information needed to thrive in the modern world" (Hirsch, 1987, p. xiii). We are shocked to see man-on-the-street interviews that reveal ignorance of common information such as the current president's name, basic geography, famous events in history, and so forth. One college student, for instance, could not give even a simple account of the Civil War, even though she had completed a high school American history course with a passing grade.

One should be concerned about what is learned in school as well as what is retained as there is certainly a core of basic information that all members of a community should know. It also seems critical, though, that students not just accumulate important facts but learn how to learn on their own. This is particularly important when students confront the complex and formal extended discourse of higher grades in school. They should then be prepared to learn later in life that which was not taught originally, or, ten years after graduation, that which has been forgotten. Professionals, parents and mentors need to engage adolescents actively in the process of becoming authentic life-time learners. There are critical elements in working with adolescents to this end.

■ CREATING A SHOULDER-TO-SHOULDER APPROACH

A shoulder-to-shoulder approach is important in a relationship between adults and adolescents to convey a sense of genuine collabo-ration. This book shows how such a partnership can be developed, including each participant's role. There is discussion of how the shoul-der-to-shoulder approach works to support better language and learn-ing. Profiles of adolescents encountered in my clinical practice are presented to serve as referents for readers to evoke their own interac-tions with adolescents. Informal, interactive diagnostic tools are also described as ways to know adolescents, to allow them to know them-selves, and to know their adult collaborators.

Interviews and questionnaires are some of the tools used to estab-lish the shoulder-to-shoulder approach. Asking students to describe their own situations using these tools conveys respect for their per-spectives and provides information not available elsewhere. Formal assessment is also discussed along with relevant diagnostic questions formulated to guide observations during testing.

■ FOSTERING ACTIVE PROBLEM SOLVING

This book stresses active problem solving in guiding students to become independent learners. The first step is to help students become aware of and to clearly define their language processing and learning needs. The informal and formal diagnostic measures are the focus in the beginning of a collaboration. Understanding their problems is nec-essary for students to appreciate the need for making plans as solu-tions. They then need to develop expertise in making appropriate, workable plans and in implementing, evaluating and revising those plans. Acquiring effective problem defining and solving ability allows adolescents to learn better now, to relearn what they may forget and enables them to teach themselves later what they have not learned. Ylvisaker and DeBonis (2000) described intervention problem solving for executive system impairments. Their approach presents the prob-lem solving process in the general format Goal–Plan–Do–Review applied within daily activities and supported by others in the life of the person in need of help. These same authors stress that "the develop-mental challenges of adolescence interact uniquely with executive sys-tem impairment to create intervention challenges requiring a flexible, collaborative and experimental approach." (p. 40) The problem solving emphasis we are attempting to describe in this book seems consistent with that of Ylvisaker and DeBonis (2000) but with an additional stress on helping adolescents identify their own problems on an ongoing basis. If adolescents do not learn to identify their own problems they will not use any strategies we teach, so this part of the process is critical. We have to engage the adolescents in the initial step in problem solving—noticing and specifying problems to be solved.

■□ CONNECTING ACADEMIC AND REAL WORLD KNOWLEDGE AND SKILLS

Discussion in this book aims to help students connect academic problem solving to that in their real lives in order to make school information relevant to their prior experience. Relevance is an important issue for most adolescents, but it is a critical issue for some. The "shadow studies" (Lounsbury & Clark, 1990; Lounsbury, & Johnston, 1985; 1988) highlighted the relevance issue. In those studies students around the country were followed and observed in a typical school day. The observers noted that much of the academic agenda in schools was irrelevant to the adolescents who were shadowed. Unless extraordinarily mature and motivated, adolescents often have difficulty integrating the abstract, sometimes dry and impersonal information of classrooms into their own experience. The school information frequently does not make sense. Although this is particularly true for adolescents with known language or learning problems, Gardner (1991) made a similar point about "successful" students. In his book, *The Unschooled Mind*, Gardner warned that many students learn what is required to earn the grade they need, but do not apply the information outside of class. Gardner cited a young woman who had successfully completed two semesters of physics at M.I.T. When included in an experiment asking her to solve a problem within a video game format, however, this successful college physics student persisted for a long period in using strategies typical of eleven year olds. Instead of applying the physics-based knowledge from her classwork that was appropriate for this game, she reverted to primitive logic (p.153).

Gardner (1991) commented that although students may accumulate information from their classes "even an ordinary degree of understanding is routinely missing in many, perhaps most students" (p.6). There is a need to ensure that school learning is comprehensible and real for students. This book suggests ways to encourage students to make connections between academic and real world thinking, to apply their natural strategies in class, and to apply their learned information out of class.

There are students who show the opposite pattern from the physics student mentioned above and fare better in the real world than in school. They solve problems and manage very well up to but not behind the schoolhouse door. Wagner (1993) referred to the tacit knowledge possessed by these kinds of students as "practical know-how," about how to manage oneself with adequate self-knowledge, how to manage others (subordinates, peers and superiors) and how to assess the practicality of an idea. This tacit knowledge was noted as a critical feature in effective managerial performance, regardless of other factors such as IQ. In our efforts to help adolescents value their out of school skills and integrate them into academics, we can identify those who already have such tacit knowledge but have not applied it in school, as well as those who struggle with practical "know how" in addition to academics.

■□ FACILITATING THE PROCESSING OF EXTENDED DISCOURSE

Language challenges differ as children advance from short conversational interchanges to reading and producing fiction and then nonfiction forms (Westby, 1985, Perera, 1986). The different style and complexity of expository language is encountered initially in fourth grade, and exposure to this kind of language increases throughout subsequent grades. Many students seem unable to progress accordingly in their language processing abilities in order to adequately manage this new kind of language. When one observes classes at various transitions in school, it is clear that many students are screened out when they are confronted with unfamiliar, abstract topics and concepts wrapped in unfamiliar, complex language. These students need help in making the leap from conversation to higher-level school language. This book suggests ways to help adolescents listen better and understand the language of class discussion and lecture, and ways of approaching the reading of novels, stories and expository chapters. A variety of strategies are discussed for helping students in comprehending paragraphs and sentences along with suggestions for coping with new vocabulary. This book aims to help those students without the inherent ability and in need of direct teaching of strategies necessary for this higher level language. Learning principles are presented to highlight effective, conscious language processing in learning.

■□ WAYS TO IMPLEMENT THE SHOULDER-TO-SHOULDER APPROACH.

Information is included for implementing the shoulder-to-shoulder, problem solving approach with various populations in varied settings within different service delivery models. Professionals working in classrooms, in college learning centers, high school resource rooms, within individual intervention settings, and collaborative or consulting relationships should find pertinent information.

One section shows the necessity of stopping to "regroup" and check adolescents' comprehension of content, of processes in learning situations and of their particular academic problems. Professionals using this approach often speak about "bridges" to new situations and this book addresses those critical times when students must be able to understand, explain and apply what they know about themselves, their strengths and weaknesses, and how they manage most effectively in a variety of situations. Students in high schools, technical school settings and rehabilitation centers can be engaged in this collaborative approach for guiding transitions to work or higher learning opportunities.

Accommodations in classrooms and workplaces will be discussed along with ways to encourage students to advocate for their own appropriate learning conditions in these settings.

■□ SUMMARY

Working effectively with adolescents for improved language and learning requires an active, honest collaboration with a shoulder-to-shoulder quality providing the "soul" of an approach that depends on mutual respect. Problem solving is fostered for involving and informing adolescents about themselves as learners. The extended discourse of academic learning requires direct teaching and guided practice in specific language strategies that are usually not in the repertoire of at risk adolescents. To appreciate the relevance of academic learning, adolescents need help in connecting their real world knowledge and natural problem solving strategies to schoolwork—to understand that they have skills that are applicable in academic settings. This shoulder-to-shoulder approach can be used with the same goals and slight variations within a variety of settings and service delivery models. Engaging adolescents in a shoulder-to-shoulder, joint problem solving effort is particularly important during transitions to higher level schooling and work. It is critical at these times that adolescents understand their own language and learning needs and the necessary accommodations that match those needs. They also need to know how to advocate for themselves to obtain the appropriate accommodations in order to do well in college or on the job.

This book includes information about how to implement the shoulder-to-shoulder, problem solving approach with various populations in varied settings within different service delivery models. Professionals working in classrooms, in college learning centers, high school resource rooms, within individual intervention settings, and collaborative or consulting relationships should find pertinent information.

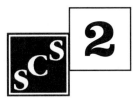

The Shoulder-to-Shoulder Approach

The potential for resistance to adult control makes a collaborative approach particularly important for adolescents. If we, as professionals or parents, are not working with adolescents, they are probably working against us or just not working at all. Andrews and Summers (1988) suggested that some adolescents seem to go directly "from the submissiveness of childhood to an aggressive 'question authority' mode of operation" (p. 70) that requires extra skill on the adult's part to help the student move beyond confrontation. If these adolescents are not actively and honestly included as a critical part of the process from beginning to end they won't engage. Many adults wouldn't either. Professionals need adolescents' information, their perspective, and their participation to be effective in helping them grow and change. Temple Grandin (1995), in her autobiographic account of her struggles with autism, complained about teachers and professionals who "wanted to discourage my weird interests and make me more normal " (p. 99). In contrast, she praised the different approach of a science teacher, Mr. Carlock, who "took my interests and used them as motivators for doing schoolwork." (p. 99). This teacher seemed to appreciate the need to collaborate with Ms. Grandin for best results.

When adolescents walk into my office, I know very little about them. I can gather information from teachers and parents or through testing, but I depend on the adolescent to fill in gaps in order to create a true picture. Adolescents have critical information, impressions, and strategies that we need to know in order to do our jobs as professionals. Establishing a shoulder-to-shoulder quality allows professionals to work with adolescents in a respectful, effective way ("It's you and I together—shoulder-to-shoulder trying to figure out how you learn best."). They have their part, we have ours, and when this shoulder-to-shoulder relationship can be developed well, effective work can be done.

In early encounters with youngsters, professionals are often preoccupied with the ideas that we bring to the session; ideas from professional reading, from meetings and seminars, from discussions with other professionals. An eagerness to "try out" these new approaches modified to fit needs revealed in diagnostic information and direct observation sometimes leaves clients in the role of simply providing opportunities for us to try new tricks.

Lucy Calkins (1991) discussed a similar phase in her early years as a writing teacher, when she spent most of her time and energy creating clever story starters to spark her students' thinking and writing. It was only later that she apparently discovered the power of helping students explore their own ideas. In an early scene from the movie, "The Dead Poets' Society," Robin Williams' character performs brilliantly in the teacher role while the students stand by passively. Later, he learns to stimulate their thinking. The view of the teacher as "star" in relationships with adolescents must be replaced if we are to foster growth and to encourage independence.

■□ STRUCTURING THE ADULT–ADOLESCENT PARTNERSHIP

I began to reflect on the client's role while observing speech-language pathology graduate students in their early therapy sessions. Their usual lessons did not seem to encourage an active role for the client or to respect the client's contribution to the process. As novices, these student speech-language pathologists were so preoccupied with materials and plans that they had difficulty attending to the client. At that time, I began examining my own style with youngsters and noticed that I often raised my volume in talking, particularly to adolescents of my height or taller. This seemed a way to establish my authority, which may have been necessary at times, but I often continued to talk in this loud voice when it was no longer necessary. This way of communicating did not foster a true collaboration.

Using Arrows

I also noticed that both the graduate students and I followed the traditional Initiation-Response-Evaluation (IRE) interactional sequence described by Cazden (1988) and referred to by Wallach and Butler (1994) as the "default pattern" for teacher-student communications in classrooms (p. 33). Everything in intervention sessions began with the clinician, then went to the student and then back to the clinician for an evaluative comment. The IRE routine was appropriate much of the time because it was the adult's responsibility in these sessions to decide certain parameters, but this way of interacting seemed to strengthen a dependence on the clinician rather than acknowledging the youngster's potential independent abilities. I struggled to express these concerns to graduate student clinicians and to show them more effective ways to relate to clients in speech language therapy. I remembered the transactional analysis model (Harris, 1969) and began to examine lessons as transactions. I explained to the students, "If all the arrows in transactions start with you, go to the client, and come back to you, it suggests that you are responsible for and necessary for all of the youngster's growth and success. This kind of interaction, if it dominates your sessions, seems to encourage a submissive role for the client and doesn't respect their abilities."

I suggested that the students try for more adult–adult transactions in their sessions by providing choices for the client, thereby encouraging active participation and personal investment in the lesson. This

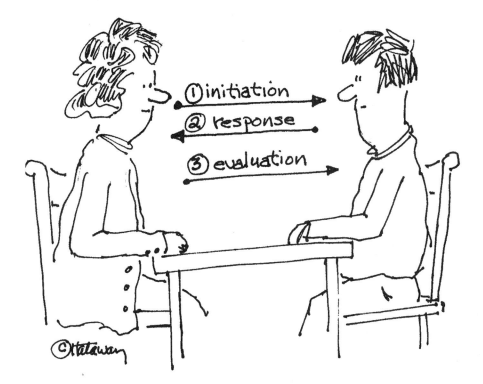

FIGURE 2-1
Using Arrows

adaptation of the transactional approach popularized by the book, "I'm OK and You're OK" (Harris, 1969) was a beginning effort to respect youngsters and to include them in their own intervention.

Building Boxes

In the evolution toward a new relationship within intervention, I next hit upon a "box-building" metaphor, in which the instructor or speech-language pathologist (SLP) in a relationship with an adolescent, builds the "box" for the youngster to grow in by creating the basic structure or boundaries of lessons. Together, then, the SLP and adolescent client establish appropriate goals, topics and specific activities providing opportunities for guided participation appropriate to the youngsters' maturity and ability. The box-building metaphor seemed not only an effective way to illustrate shared responsibility within a therapeutic or teaching/learning relationship but also to define the parent-child relationship.

If the box constructed by the parent or clinician is too large and flexible, the child may be given inappropriate responsibility for decision making. They might be asked to decide things that they do not have the skills or maturity to decide, and this can hinder growth. If the box is too confining, the child's role may be to simply comply with adult direction. Again, there will be limited opportunities to grow. The challenge is to design a "box" so that an adult can be accountable and responsible in guiding a youngster's growth but still allow for active contribution from the youngster with an appropriate balance between choice and guidance.

■□ DEVELOPING A SHOULDER-TO-SHOULDER STRUCTURE

Having drawn arrows and boxes, I was still not satisfied with the characterization of a teaching/learning relationship that seemed most respectful of clients, especially adolescents, in their own intervention. As I worked with more and more adolescents, I began to think of a "shoulder-to-shoulder" interaction, in which the adolescent and adult, side-by-side, consider and try to understand the client's language and learning, his or her strengths and weaknesses with the purpose of developing appropriate personalized plans and strategies. In this way, the adolescent and adult could build the diagnostic and intervention sessions together.

It is interesting that Prendeville (1991) described similar roles for very young children, who, as participants in a conversation, create that conversation together. Prendeville stressed that these children were not simply alternating in the talker–listener roles, but were contributing to and shaping a conversation together.

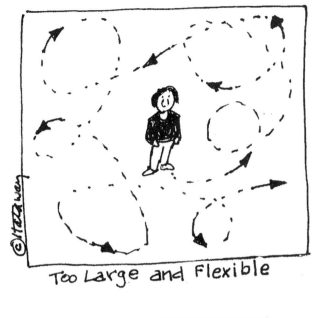

Too Large and Flexible

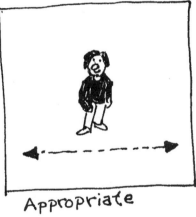

Appropriate

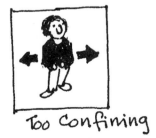

Too Confining

FIGURE 2-2
Building Boxes

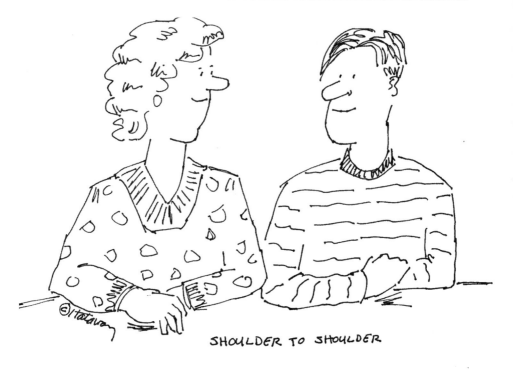

SHOULDER TO SHOULDER

FIGURE 2-3
Shoulder-to-Shoulder

This shoulder-to-shoulder collaboration seems to characterize a desired relationship for professionals working with adolescents. In this stance, shoulder-to-shoulder, the role of the clinician, teacher, special educator, vocational counselor, and so forth. is to respect what only the adolescent can contribute. Their perspectives, insights, specific experiences, feelings, and evaluations provide information that cannot be obtained in any other way. Without this contribution, the professionals cannot do their part in guiding creative planning, and utilizing skills, information and insight appropriately for each adolescent.

Delineating the Adult's Role

As adults and responsible professionals, we need to create an environment that allows for collaboration *with* adolescents. We have to ask the right questions, make observations, encourage and expand youngsters' comments, set an adult-to-adult tone, a "we're in this together" attitude, a shoulder-to-shoulder approach. How? By having respect for the unique information and perspective of the adolescent, by realizing that we cannot apply our skills to clients like Band-Aids, and by appreciating that adolescents can inform our work. We have to be alert to what we can learn from adolescents, what they have either figured out about their own language and learning or what they can reveal that will allow us to figure it out together. Andrews and Summers (1988) in discussing their work with adolescents in voice therapy suggested ways clinicians can respond to facilitate responses. Their suggestions included paraphrasing, reflecting the feelings behind statements made by adolescents, clarifying information and feelings, making tentative inferences, and affirming the comments.

We need, as the adult collaborator, to downplay our own "performance" in order to be better listeners and observers. We can observe our clients' conversational skills, language and articulation, their right-wrong answers and vocabulary use, of course, but we need also to engage them in meta-discussions, in describing their experiences, their ways of proceeding, so we can learn and plan well together. We can select a variety of tools for eliciting the adolescents' information.

Utilizing Tools

The learning interview (see Chapter 5) has been one specific tool that helps to introduce the shoulder-to-shoulder structure. The questions in the interview are authentic—this is not a test and the interviewer does not know the answers. The questions open up discussion and lead to personal reporting about students' own experience. Often my student's comments within this interview have suggested recommendations and plans that I would not have formulated on my own.

For instance, I have learned which questions sprinkled through the interview reveal a pattern of difficulty with sustained listening. In describing their teachers, students complain about those who "just talk and talk," or "just give us notes to copy" as contrasted with favorite teachers who are "fun" or "funny." When asked how they manage when they are bored in class and what they do to stay attentive at these times, adolescents often seem at a loss, at the mercy of luck because they don't know what to do when they do not have an engaging "fun" teacher.

These problems in sustained listening suggest a need for planning, with the student, to recognize when they are becoming bored and to develop specific attending strategies for those situations. Shared information in the interview guides such joint planning. Encouraging students to evaluate the adult's observations and suggestions ("I think you are having difficulty with these kinds of situations—when the teacher talks for a long time? Does this sound right to you? Am I on the right track?") is another way to show that you value the student's part in building the intervention plan. The shoulder-to-shoulder quality is figurative of course ("It's you and I together, shoulder-to-shoulder, getting your language and learning out here for us to observe ... "), because the eye contact that comes from genuine joint exploration and planning is important. One needs to maintain a face-to-face posture as you meet shoulder-to-shoulder with adolescents.

Another way to establish and maintain this relationship is to discuss youngsters' current school assignments to uncover specific problems and to target goals. In such contexts, adolescents have the opportunity to explain their assignments and to respond to genuine clarification questions; to explain what is easy and hard for them in specific assignments; to share typical difficulties they have with frequently assigned tasks; and to discuss their usual ways of solving these problems.

With the insights elicited by the learning interview and discussion of specific school assignments as a base, the educator and adolescent can then discuss formal diagnostic findings regarding language and learning needs. The adult is better able to present the formal test results after adolescents have had the first opportunity to define themselves through their own reports. Adolescents might better appreciate test findings presented in relation to prior discussion based on their own observations. With information gathered informally and throughout testing they can target specific goals and make plans for intervention with the adult's suggesting appropriate materials and strategies for further discovery and practice. The collaborators can return, regularly, to the students' school work to integrate new strategies into assignments and to uncover other problems to be attacked or spontaneous strengths to be utilized consciously.

Modeling Effective Learning

When students explain their assignments and learning/study processes, their adult collaborator can model the heuristic style of an effective learner, the "wrinkled brow" that characterizes the very necessary questions and disequilibrium that are visible, audible signs of learning. The adult can comment on this learner style as a good one for learners of all ages (not just adolescents with language and learning problems). In this way they can emphasize that real learning includes confusion and questioning which lead to specific attention and problem solving.

This is an important aspect of the adult's role in the shoulder-to-shoulder collaborations—to model active learning and to discuss it when it occurs, to make the implicit process of learning explicit for adolescents who may not notice on their own these characteristics of communication and learning. With this modeling and discussing, different aspects of language, communication, and learning can become relevant for students. These discoveries often become shared "private jokes" that reoccur within the collaboration.

For instance, one high school senior demonstrated overprediction, as a favored approach to school reading assignments, that is, she seemed to rely on her own experience or logic without reading closely to confirm her assumptions. This student was a better predictor than confirmer (Goodman & Burke, 1972). I noted this tendency in this young adolescent client and explained that it is effective to use prior experience in approaching a lesson saying, "You should always use what you know rather than 'reinventing the wheel' every day." I also suggested that she needed to add another strategy, checking with the text for verification of her ideas. After understanding both effective use of old information and her less effective overprediction in repeated examples, this young woman began to "catch" herself overpredicting. When that occurred, we would both appreciate this as typical of her style. These discoveries and comments were not reprimands or criticisms and were often couched as questions. "It seems to me that you are predicting based on your own experience in this instance, but forgot to check to see if your prediction worked. Do you think this is what happened?" As the adult observer of this student's learning, I needed to check my assumptions with these kinds of questions in the same way that this student needed to check her reading predictions. I also needed to reassure the student that information we discovered would remain confidential and that it would not be used against a student (Andrews & Summers, 1988), that she would not have more than the usual points taken off for an impulsive response, for instance, just because this was a current goal and she should "know better."

Students are not threatened by these observations when the shoulder-to-shoulder approach has been established as a joint discover-and-discuss process, especially as I include observations about my own way of processing. I inadvertently demonstrate some of the same strategies at times, such as overpredicting without checking, and I am always delighted when this occurs naturally because it proves that the student's behavior is not a "deficit," although it may occur more often than it should. Students begin to appreciate that their strategies or answers to questions may be logical and good even though they have not yet reached the "right" answer, that everyone must actively process when learning, and that one rarely automatically understands new concepts. Many adolescents persist in viewing learning as already knowing rather than appreciating that everyone struggles to learn some things at some times, and that quick answers are not forthcoming or even desirable for all questions. Adults need to make this aspect of learning very clear in order to keep adolescents in the learning game. Otherwise they may continue to give up at the first stumbling block, assuming that all is lost when they do not conceptualize quickly.

Delineating the Adolescent's Role

The adolescent's role in this shoulder-to-shoulder arrangement includes describing and reporting real world examples from his or her experience to use in language and learning exercises. When they provide the content for discussions, the work takes on relevance. The student observes, monitors his or her language and learning and learns about him or herself as a learner. The student identifies specific strengths and problem areas, makes collaborative plans, and refines those plans with the guidance and active collaboration of an adult. The adolescent provides the content; the adult sets the tone and structure (the box); and together they work to build each session and to effect growth in the adolescent's language and learning. In this process, the student practices a variety of communication skills focused on problem solving.

Practicing and Developing Language

The adolescent in this collaboration provides an ongoing sample of linguistic ability gathered in discussions that require the reporting of events, identifying problems, and discussing and evaluating plans with appropriate vocabulary and use of elaborated language designed to make their information clear to the adult. Adolescents have authentic reasons to expand their linguistic skills with the help of the SLP in order to communicate exactly what they mean within this relationship. They should learn to clarify what they know and feel in their attempts to explain. They learn, with modeling and direct teaching, to ask effective questions to better understand their collaborative partner's comments and suggestions. This shoulder-to-shoulder approach requires the student to use language within intervention settings in the purposeful effort to find and solve problems. This can certainly stimulate discovery of and extension of world knowledge, (schemata, categories and inferences), pragmatic knowledge (intent, listener awareness, topic management, response to contextual variation, (identifying and repairing conversational breakdowns) and discourse knowledge (scripts, story grammar, text cohesion). The construction of knowledge comes within the context of oral explanations of events, diagnostic findings and ongoing discussion of specific school assignments.

Using Strategies for and Reflecting on Extended Discourse

Finally, the student works at and gains competence in managing and using higher-level communication that is important for adolescents. Elaborated utterances are necessary for the shoulder-to-shoulder, problem solving approach and can be taught through this collaboration. It has been suggested that adolescents need to be taught strategies for learning rather than just content (Nelson, 1998; Lord-Larson and McKinley, 1995) and this approach provides a context for teaching strategies and for enhancing meta-awareness of the strategies taught. The adolescents' responsibility for and increasing ability to reflect on learning problems, to predict the efficacy of joint plans and to evaluate results are critical to this process and reflect growth in metacognitive and metapragmatic language skills. Therefore, the adolescent's role includes learning how to reflect on language and learning during the problem solving process.

Satisfying Conditions of Quality Work

The validity of this approach is supported by its consistency with other descriptions of best practices. For instance, Glasser's (1993a) six conditions of quality work within a classroom are consistent with the collaborative, shoulder-to-shoulder approach with adolescents. In order to elicit students' best efforts and best work, Glasser suggested, first, that students must know the educator as a person and appreciate the educator's role in providing a caring environment for work. Second, students must believe that the work the educator engages them in is useful. Third, the students must be willing to put significant effort into what they do, that is, "to do the best they can do" (p. 23). Fourth, the students must learn to evaluate their own work and to improve it. Glasser notes that students usually know what quality work is but do not associate quality work with schools. Glasser's fifth and sixth conditions are that "quality work always feels good" (p. 24) and is never destructive.

It seems that the shoulder-to-shoulder approach can satisfy these six conditions for quality work. First, it allows students to get to know their collaborator as a person and co-learner through the discussion of problems, strategies and solutions. Second, it helps them to see the validity of assignments when they have been "in on it" from the beginning. Third, adolescent partners in this collaborative approach are more willing to put good effort into plans because of their investment, the personalizing of the process and the support of their collaborator. Fourth, the ongoing joint discussion and evaluation during problem solving provides a model of the self-evaluation one hopes will result. Fifth, this kind of collaboration, when it works well, should feel good to both partners. Finally, the more one works actively with adolescents on their behalf, the more real and "quality" that work feels.

Feeney and Ylvisaker (1995) described three adolescents who had been or were in danger of being expelled from their schools. A review of the students' daily experience in school revealed that their academic work required organization and planning skills beyond their ability and that they seldom had success; that the students had no control over what kind, how or when they did their work; and that punishment had increased their negative behavior. These students clearly did not see their work as quality work. A problem solving approach that seemed consistent with Glasser's conditions for quality work and with the intent of the shoulder-to-shoulder approach was implemented and resulted in improved school performance for these three students.

◼◻ IMPLEMENTING THE APPROACH IN CLASSROOMS

Establishing a shoulder-to-shoulder, problem solving approach within small groups or larger classes presents different challenges from those presented in paired relationships, but it can be done. For instance, the learning interview can be completed and then discussed in class to encourage the appreciation of differences in learning style and language processing and to allow for group problem solving in order to accommodate differences. One teacher might be a fast mover and talker, who is comfortable covering new material quickly. Another teacher might favor a cycling approach and introduce information without expecting mastery on the first encounter knowing that the class will return to the concept later. Either of these instructional styles may cause serious difficulty for the sequential learner who wants to understand new concepts thoroughly before moving on, and who finds it difficult to process at such a fast rate. These issues can be revealed in responses to the learning interview. In group problem solving sessions, students might request more time for discussing new information before the instructor moves on, might ask for more frequent and clear "stopping" places for clarifying and questioning new concepts or procedures, and/or the teacher might decide to write key words or phrases on the board or on an overhead transparency to guide student's understanding and to slow down the pace of presentation.

Students might find kindred spirits through this kind of group problem solving discussion, those who identify the same problems and can offer new solutions. They might be surprised that even successful students have problems in processing. Teachers who utilize cooperative learning can involve students in planning alternative ways to learn the same materials, include them in evaluation of the process, and encourage discussion of problems encountered in specific lessons along with discussions of how students resolved their dilemmas. Professionals working with peers regularly engage in joint problem solving and collaborative goal setting (Nelson, 1998) and can encourage this same approach within adolescent groups. Teachers in this shoulder-to-shoulder stance with students do not, of course, relinquish the decisions appropriate to their role in guiding learning, but include students in the process of creating a classroom environment that facilitates learning. Students who have not felt a part of a class before might be able to participate in this kind of effort.

Planning S.P.A.C.E.D. Lessons

Mini-lessons can be used as a format for introducing strategies in the problem solving approach. To guide teachers in planning effective lessons, I developed a procedure with the acronym, SPACED (Tattershall, 1994a). The teacher evokes the students' schemas (S) pertinent to a new topic, includes a problem solving (P) element, elicits active (A) participation of students to ensure best attention, makes the important points very clear (C), provides many examples (E) for the new point or concept, often elicited from students, and finally, reviews the lesson by discussing (D) problems encountered and solutions students devised as they tried to understand the concepts. SPACED lessons organized in this way contribute to a shoulder-to-shoulder atmosphere in classrooms by providing opportunities for students to reflect on their learning and to gain ownership of their specific problems during lessons. The structure also provides discussion of solutions personalized for and by students. The discussion of the learning that occurs within lessons is critical for adolescents not naturally talented in the problem solving necessary for learning. By regularly hearing others discuss problems that occurred in a particular homework assignment, for instance, the adolescent with learning problems begins to appreciate that everyone has difficulty in learning at times and that there are a variety of ways to solve learning problems. The C (be clear) emphasizes the need to narrow the focus of a lesson to one or two points for better learning and also models the importance of being specific in identifying problems. Providing extra examples is extremely helpful for those with language learning difficulty who typically need many, varied examples before clearly understanding a new concept and better understand when the examples are explained in the language of peers.

Predicting Grades

In the interest of engaging her students actively in the learning process within a middle school health class, one classroom teacher added a grade prediction component to her unit tests. This teacher provided a box at the bottom of the test listing the possible letter grades and the point ranges for each letter grade. She asked students to check the grade range they thought they would receive on the test and they were rewarded with extra points on the test if they accurately predicted their grade. This seemed like an effective way to engage students in their own learning within a typical classroom procedure. This teacher later refined the idea by asking students not only to guess their overall grade, but to indicate with small dots those answers that might be wrong (the dot system). This seemed helpful in directing students' attention to their specific knowledge and could easily be extended to homework assignments. If students were required to identify, specifically, what they did not understand in their daily work, they could then be engaged in developing alternative ways to learn difficult concepts. In these ways, this teacher created opportunities for students to know themselves as learners in addition to their learning the facts required for the health test.

Predicting Questions

In the effort to engage students in their own learning, many teachers have invited students to predict and list possible test questions about content material. This assignment seems to direct students to reflect on the teacher's and textbook author's signaling of important information in order to select questions that might be asked. The next day's discussion of the questions and students' reasons for focusing on certain topics or facts ("That's an interesting question. Why did you decide on that one?") is an excellent way to actively include students in their own learning. It allows those with less effective language processing to acquire skills for creating questions and provides insight to teachers about their students' approaches to learning.

Evaluating Materials and Activities

Teachers can also include students in evaluating textbooks, test types, and different ways of teaching or learning. Students can preview books at the beginning of each semester, identify potential problems (too many big words, few pictures, too many charts, a lot of dates to remember) and discuss strategies for coping with those problems. Teachers can offer a choice of various test formats and require students to explain their choices. Students can be guided in rewriting test questions in their own style and to contrast their version with the original, for example, by showing or explaining why their way is better. Teachers can model a variety of ways to present and learn material followed by students implementing various approaches in small groups and evaluations of the various strategies.

Various ways to value the students' point of view and include them actively in their own learning are presented. Problem solving becomes the vehicle for the collaboration in most instances. The teachers do not relinquish responsibility and simply let students plan the curriculum. Instead they include students in evaluating in order to create opportunities to problem solve and perhaps vary the classroom plans. Students and teachers, for instance, may agree that a textbook is difficult because of convoluted writing but they have to find ways in joint planning to use that book effectively in order to learn. Including students in these kinds of shoulder-to-shoulder efforts illustrates how to deal practically with real, ongoing learning problems, to include students in the process, and to make plans side-by-side with adolescents.

■□ SUMMARY

The shoulder-to-shoulder quality, the "soul" of an effective relationship with adolescents, requires both partners to value the information and observations contributed to the collaboration. Adult partners particularly need to appreciate the importance of adolescents' points of view as the starting point for gathering information about them. Further, at risk youngsters need to feel more competent and to have control in some of the decisions affecting them.

The shoulder-to-shoulder stance evolved as an appropriate structure for productive joint problem solving in which adults and adolescents have particular roles. The adults set the tone for mutual respect using tools such as interviews, questionnaires, discussion of school assignments, and modeling of active learning. The adolescents provide the content and issues for discussion and present their language needs and own observations to guide the joint planning. This process of sharing information and observations fosters "meta" skills necessary for adolescents to progress beyond basic levels of functioning. The shoulder-to-shoulder quality in the problem solving process seems to satisfy the conditions for quality work (Glasser, 1993a) necessary for adults and adolescents to have an investment in what they do together. Teachers and SLPs can implement this approach in classrooms and therapy settings by using the learning interview, practicing strategies with cooperative learning, planning SPACED lessons that allow discussion of the learning process, and utilizing student predictions of grades and test questions. Using the problem solving process, students are actively engaged in identifying problems as well as making plans and implementing them within these classroom learning activities.

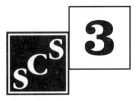

The Active Problem Solving Approach

Problem solving is what effective adults do in life. It is the goal of this book to show how to teach adolescents to problem solve more consciously and effectively and to show professionals how to do the same in our work with adolescents. The intention is to help adolescents become full, active partners in the shoulder-to-shoulder approach through joint problem solving. Given the tool of effective problem defining and solving, adolescents can relearn specific school information or teach themselves what they never really learned—how to become lifelong learners.

Bransford (1993) described traditional "transmission" approaches in education which presumed that just telling or "passing on" knowledge was effective. Many adolescents have failed in these kinds of classes because of poor memories—the information they were supposed to acquire directly was not understood or stored by simply listening and looking. Others have succeeded in the short term merely by memorizing facts transmitted but without understanding. Both groups need an alternative, more effective way to learn. Active problem solving offers one solution. Bransford (1993) suggested that working through examples and sample problems is critical for learning, a strategy that should work well when the sample problems are personally relevant to adolescents, particularly when these problems are impeding their success in school. Rapid changes in the world require powerful thinking and learning skills (Resnick, 1987) and an emphasis on active problem solving seems appropriate for exercising these skills.

In the effort to foster problem solving, students are guided in developing a systematic way of identifying problems, of deciding whether they are potentially solvable, and, in the process, becoming aware of "aspects of their knowledge that they otherwise might not consider on their own" (Bransford, 1993, p.185). Students with tacit knowledge (Wagner, 1993) can, through problem solving in school, become conscious of their real world abilities applicable to school learning. The intent is to help adolescents solve their immediate school learning problems and also acquire independent effective problem solving skills that can be generalized to many situations including school learning.

■□ INVOLVING ADOLESCENTS IN PROBLEM SOLVING

Speech-language pathologists and others engaged in diagnostic-through-intervention efforts have always worked within a problem solving framework. However, clinicians have not always actively engaged clients in the process from beginning to end. As professionals, we have identified the problems, created possible solutions, and then guided clients to follow our recommendations. One wonders how much students retain after the ten year span cited by the comedian in the beginning of this book if the adult partner has taken most of the responsibility and the students have not been active from the outset. A more collaborative arrangement can benefit adolescents who want to become independent learners but lack the tools to do so. A joint problem solving approach for defining and resolving language and learning difficulties provides adolescents with tools for independent learning. Strategies for assisting students in acquiring those tools form the essence of this book.

■□ PROVIDING A VEHICLE FOR COMMUNICATION

Besides helping to resolve immediate difficulties, problem solving can become a vehicle for more effective communication with adolescents. By creating a shared focus on adolescents' problems and valuing their input or point of view, collaborating adults gain the adolescents' attention and facilitate communication. Adolescents need to discuss and expand their explanations to clarify problems or to present possible solutions. They give reasons for their conclusions rather than just commenting in short, simple sentences. They compare ideas particularly when devising plans for solving problems. Adults are not "fixing" adolescents in this process, they are working together with them. The very nature of adolescence makes this approach particularly important because it addresses the need at this time in life for appreciation and respect while contributing to adolescents' developing understanding of their power, their ability, and their concept of themselves.

AVOIDING BIASES IN PROBLEM SOLVING

Wagner (1993) described common biases that affected rational problem solving of managers in business that seem relevant to interactions between educators and adolescents. These biases include:

1. Overestimating the frequency of highly salient events over the less well known;
2. Giving more weight to information received early than to later information;
3. Discovering what one expected to discover;
4. Noting total number of successes without appreciating the ratio of success to total number of experiences;
5. Focusing on the concrete more than on abstract information;
6. Applying evaluative criteria inconsistently;
7. Not changing formed opinions;
8. Persisting in using a strategy that has been, but is no longer appropriate; and
9. Overestimating the stability of data based on small samples.

It is important to recognize and avoid these biases in our experiences with adolescents. The label "adolescent" for instance, comes with assumed characteristics—rebellious, stubborn, know-it-all—that often prevent an uncluttered view of clients at this age. The impressions of teachers and parents appearing in written or oral reports can evoke opinions before even meeting young clients. To get beyond the obvious, to avoid the glare of untested assumptions, and to have a fresh start with adolescents, it helps to concentrate on learning from the adolescents themselves. One should not "reinvent the wheel" by ignoring the reports of others but the focus should be on what adolescents actually know or can show about their language abilities and learning.

One middle school student skipped class and lied repeatedly creating a bad first impression on his teachers. Fortunately, his parents went into action and he was enrolled in counseling. This youngster began to appreciate the need to change his behavior and was apparently making progress when I was called in to test him. I sent him to inform teachers that he would be out of class for the testing, and he came back in tears because his teachers did not believe his excuse for missing class! This was understandable based on his behavioral history, but the lesson this young boy learned about first impressions was painful.

Professionals have to fight the tendency to "imprint" on first bits of information and keep their minds open while working together with adolescents. Otherwise, the professional's bias may mask emerging abilities, problems, or experiences that have not been a part of the previous record. Troubled adolescents particularly need a clean slate to allow the uncovering of previously unrecognized strengths useful in supporting known weaknesses.

An understandable tendency of adults leads us to overdo our encouragement of adolescents who have had little success. We sometimes insult them by doing so because they know that the ratio of their successes to total number of experiences is still heavily weighted toward failure. One youngster with serious reading and writing problems was not impressed, for example, by a teacher's praise of his dictated writing. In her attempt to encourage him, the teacher was overly effusive in her comments about his potential as a writer, and his reaction was "She has pipe dreams!" The same issue arose with a severely dyslexic adolescent girl whose parents were desperately looking for ways to raise her self-esteem. Unfortunately, they chose to praise her for tasks that, in her view, were not praiseworthy and she felt patronized rather than encouraged. Realistic and honest appraisals show respect for the adolescent as a partner and prevent this pitfall in problem solving.

Adolescents can fall prey to the bias of overconfidence based on recent successes and not appreciate that their total record is still seriously unsuccessful. Some youngsters have no systematic way to judge the parts (each grade) in relation to the whole (the semester average). Their problem solving can be adversely affected when they note only concrete aspects of a situation ("Well I asked for help!") without appreciation of subtle, abstract factors ("It may have been the way you asked rather than the actual words you said."). We need to consider in our collaborating with students, the standard scores and grades as concrete information that can reveal problems. At the same time, we can help students notice and value their effective strategies, attitudes and out of school success experiences as more abstract evidence of their potential as learners. We need to help adolescents notice nonverbal signs of teacher disapproval of specific acts and to appreciate the cumulative effect of these acts on teacher attitudes toward their students, that is, to help adolescents think beyond specific visual or auditory experiences to the more abstract level of communication.

The youngster who remembers one recent good grade, often "rides" on that grade without considering the effect of a subsequent low grade. This student is falling prey to bias based on a small sample. The student who focuses on the problem areas of academics and gives no credence to successes in nonacademic domains is applying an inconsistent criterion to good work. The need to be clear about data, to discuss findings aloud, to check understandings by having adolescents explain their thinking at various points in the problem solving process are necessary strategies for avoiding biases.

One other concern must be considered as a pitfall in problem solving. This is the tendency for "wishful thinking" and/or overestimating the potency of one's actions. Students are often unrealistic in their vocational goals in view of their limitations in related skills. The disorganized adolescent often assumes that having the intention of doing better will cause success although this student may have no specific plan for achieving improved results. If adolescents are going to progress beyond wishful thinking, adult partners have to intervene to cause realistic self-appraisal of abilities and ensure that students make specific, effective plans for achieving goals.

◼□ HELPING ADOLESCENTS IDENTIFY SPECIFIC PROBLEMS

Professionals encounter one group of adolescents who do not identify specific problems they have, and also know little about their strengths. They present with a vague, general feeling of *dis*-ease about themselves as learners but without a clear understanding that might lead to solutions. This group seems to assume that all their academic problems are attributable to the label they have been assigned (whether it is learning disability, attention-deficit, language disordered, slow learner, lower track, etc.) and that, because they have this label, nothing can be done to change their performance. Bransford and Stein (1984) suggested that many people assume that problems are simply "facts of life" (p. 12) and accept them as such without really noting them as problems. They also described a "let me out of here" (p. 4) avoidance response of those with limited tolerance for problems. There is also the issue of "courage span" or how long one can face his or her problems without feeling bad (Wertime, 1979). Some adolescents who do not define problems may be inattentive for these reasons.

Although some of these same adolescents may demonstrate good problem solving outside of school, they do not apply this natural skill in school, perhaps because they think diagnostic labels determine their school success. Their comments suggest that school learning is completely different from other experiences and is dependent on a talent or magical gift that was handed out at birth, but not to them. One young woman declared during testing, "I give up quickly because I either know it or I don't." In other words, she did not have the gift for automatically producing answers. Because of these apparent misconceptions, this group of youngsters does not even begin to problem solve for school by identifying specific problems that might be solvable.

This group of adolescents obviously needs help in identifying specific problems as the first step in problem solving for better learning. Engaging them in learning interviews, completing questionnaires or checklists of typical learning problems and discussing findings from formal diagnostic testing may help them pinpoint their learning problems. Modeling the process of clarifying, then narrowing, problems to be addressed is necessary for this group of youngsters. They need guided experience in monitoring their understanding of what they hear and read in school to identify specific concepts, assignments, questions, and vocabulary they do not understand. Those students who neglect detail when listening or reading, for example, will profit from "proof-listening" activities in which they tape their oral reading and then listen as they silently reread the material. Students can discover through this proof-listening, what they typically do when they read—their usual reading miscue types. Instructors in this kind of collaborative effort, might listen to students' reading, identify miscues, tell students how many and what kind of miscues to listen for in their proof-listening to direct their attention. Knowing the total number and discovering the usual kinds of errors they make can help students better know themselves as readers and can guide their independent proof-reading. A record showing the students' accuracy in proofreading or proof-listening as compared with that of the adult collaborator can document improvement in identifying specific reading problems within these exercises.

With the same goal of helping students identify specific learning problems, teachers can check listening comprehension by routinely asking students after lectures or discussion to restate new concepts in their own words. Students' attempts to paraphrase their teachers' explanations can reveal ongoing language processing problems that occur within classroom learning. Some students might, for instance, respond impulsively within discussions without appropriate reflection. The adult in the collaboration can identify this problem to the student ("You seemed to leap to a creative idea, one that related in part to what has been discussed, but your idea did not fit *all* the facts."). Ideally, this student would be encouraged to use this creativity and spontaneity in brainstorming exercises, but be guided in supporting assertions with facts as needed and in recognizing when to apply these two different approaches.

Problems such as impulsive responding within class discussions or writing assignments can be noted and counted to enhance awareness of another kind of specific, recurring problem. Students can also discuss the Checklist of Study Problems (see Box 3–1), keep track of those study probems that are pertinent, and add to this list as new problems are revealed within school assignments. Students can be required to specify their problems when they request help or clarification. Teachers can respond to requests with a "You first, then me" approach in which the teacher says, "You tell me what you think first, even if you only know a little bit. Then I will help." This response requires students to go beyond just appreciating that they are confused and to become specific and clear about their particular difficulty. This can save time for both teachers and students. Students who become proficient at clarifying their problems and stating them specifically are practicing a skill that will help in school and will also make them more effective employees. If they approach their boss by first explaining a problem specifically, and telling what they think first, this will save time and facilitate the problem solving on the job. Anecdotes that equate this skill to employee–employer communication might make this meaningful for adolescents to practice in school.

BOX 3–1: *Checklist of Study Problems*

Check the comments below that are true for you. Double check those that are typical problems for you. Add other study problems you have.

1. You did an assignment wrong because you did not hear the teacher's instructions.
2. You completed your work quickly and did not check for errors.
3. Your teacher got mad at you and you did not know why.
4. You did not write down all your assignment.
5. You left your book at school and needed it for homework.
6. You received a bad grade because you did not read the directions.
7. You read an assignment but did not remember what you read.
8. You studied, thought you knew the material at home, but did not do well on the test.
9. You did your homework but left it at home or lost it.
10. You got a bad grade on a test because you did not finish.
11. You do not have a regular study time. You study only for tests.
12. You can repeat what the teacher said, but you often do not understand.
13. You do not have a place to write homework assignments down.
14. You often do not raise your hand even when you know the answer because you are afraid you'll be wrong.

Teachers can cause students to evaluate what they know and do not know in order to identify problems at test-taking time. Students can be required to predict their grade on a test and, more specifically, to mark with a "dot" those questions that they found difficult. To reinforce this active problem identifying in test taking, teachers can reward students with extra credit for accurately predicting their grade and/or for knowing which of their answers might be wrong (their dots). If students become aware of and accurate in identifying what they do not know on tests, they can be guided in using this same approach to studying before the test. They can identify the problems, that is, what they do not understand or readily recall and then study those specific items more thoroughly. Knowing what they need to study, and identifying the problems, leads to better independent learning.

Teachers can also encourage problem identification by requiring students to label assigned tasks or parts of tasks using a traffic light analogy: Red (I do not know this and will probably need help to understand it.); Yellow (I recognize this but am not really sure. However, I may be able to do this with extra effort and time. I am learning this.); or Green (I know this well and can do it by myself without too much effort or time.) Using a traffic light analogy, include students in evaluating their learning on a regular basis, engage them in thinking about what they know and don't know, and provide time for discussing problems with school assignments to provide opportunities for students to gain skill in the problem solving process.

Bransford and Stein (1984) stressed the importance of identifying problems. In a project Bransford guided in a business consultation, he assigned all workers, from top executives to those in low paid positions, the task of listing problems that they observed in the company over a period of several weeks. This seemed somewhat unusual in the business setting where workers often minimize problems to seem competent and/or to avoid being considered a complainer. In this case, however, the exercise proved effective in introducing and establishing the importance of identifying problems as the first part of the problem solving process for improving the business.

This project of finding problems has important implications for school learning. In the interest of helping students quickly, professionals sometimes teach needed strategies or provide solutions without having students first identify problems. When students do not identify their problems themselves, there is always the risk that they will not apply the strategies taught in class. For instance, students often recognize the strategy of creating a mnemonic by spelling a word using the first letters of words or phrases they need to store. They will comment that a teacher had once suggested this plan for remembering a specific fact or set of facts (HOMES to recall the names of the Great Lakes). They seem to have left this plan with that particular teacher and that particular project rather than incorporate it into their own strategies for solving real problems they later identify.

Word problems in math provide another example of teachers' skipping the problem identifying and going directly to teaching strategies for solving problems. Students are rarely invited to identify real world problems to be presented as word problems in math class. If students are involved in identifying their problems in learning, they might find the process more relevant and use strategies taught when needed.

Box 3–2, Ways to Encourage Students to Identify Problems, delineates these and other ways of encouraging students to identify problems. It includes references to pages or sections in the text where each strategy is addressed.

■❑ HELPING ADOLESCENTS MAKE PLANS

A second group of adolescents can be surprisingly good at describing their academic problems, but they do not try to find solutions or make

---

BOX 3–2: *Ways to Encourage Students to Identify Problems*

1. Learning interview (Chapter 5).
2. Homework questionnaires (Chapter 5).
3. Students' paraphrasing teachers' concepts (Chapter 3).
4. Discussion of problems in homework assignments (Chapter 3).
5. Students' predicting grades and using the "dot system" on tests (Chapter 2).
6. Proofreading and proof-listening activities (Chapter 3).
7. Students indicate level of difficulty of tasks, problems, test questions using the traffic light colors (Chapter 3).
8. Teachers use the "You first and then me" response to requests for help (Chapter 3).
9. Discovering, listing and discussing problems that occur in classroom learning (Chapter 3).
10. Modeling and eliciting real world word problems for math (Chapter 3).

---

plans. It is important to find out why such adolescents do not try to solve problems they identify. They may, for example, hold the assumptions described above that learning is a talent given to others or that the identified problems are to be expected with learning disabilities, attention problems, or whatever label they have been given, and that nothing can be done. In attempts to explain the diagnostic labels or in advocating for adolescents with learning problems, professionals need to be careful about giving the impression that these labels are "lifetime sentences" that override all solutions. Adolescents need to understand that the label they have been given can explain why they are having a particular learning problem, but that identifying a specific problem and the reason for it is just the beginning. They need to find solutions— to go beyond defining school learning problems to making plans. In this effort, students need guidance in recognizing their natural use of problem solving strategies outside of school. For example, teenagers do not abandon a disabled car on a major highway, assuming that nothing can be done, even if this is a chronic problem presented by this car. Just as they make plans to solve a particular car problem (call a parent or friend, call a tow truck ...), they must make plans to solve learning problems when they occur. One can introduce the idea of creating plans by providing recommended plans for identified problems (see Box 3–3, Plans For Study Problems). Students can match plans to problems previously identified in their Checklist of Study Problems (Box 3–1), tell why a particular plan seems to best fit their needs and discuss other possible plans. Teachers should be alert for opportunities to note and reinforce plans or solutions that students create in response to

BOX 3–3: *Plans for Study Problems*

Instructions for students: Match each plan below to its corresponding problem on the Checklist Of Study Problems (Box 3–1). Write the appropriate number for the problem on each line.

____ **a.** "Could you explain that a different way? I'm confused."

____ **b.** Try to find your errors first, then have someone else check. See how many you were able to find on your own.

____ **c.** Use the "Two Thumbs" approach. Cover the directions, look, predict, and then check-check.

____ **d.** Ask someone else what you did that made her mad. Don't do that again.

____ **e.** Use a "home locker" and a homework folder for all homework.

____ **f.** Know where, when and how the teacher usually gives directions. Be ready.

____ **g.** Use the "dot" system for tests. Don't skip questions— guess the hard ones. You can come back if you have time.

____ **h.** Warm up by looking through the chapter first. Make a web to show title and subtitles, then read each section stopping to make a note after each section.

____ **i.** Take your assignment book to your locker after school to know what materials you will need for homework.

____ **j.** Test yourself after you study to see what really "stuck" in your brain. Study the information that did not stick the first time.

____ **k.** Make a reward system for every time you study at your scheduled time.

____ **l.** Start your answer with "I'm not sure but ..." and make a good guess.

homework problem. Listing strategies for reference by others might encourage students' awareness and valuing of their own problem solving.

Helping Adolescents Evaluate and Improve Plans

There are adolescents who have academic difficulties but identify their problems relatively well and also try to make plans. Unfortunately, they often create ineffective plans that are grandiose or impractical, given their skills or personalities. Their plans sometimes reflect good intentions without a specific set of actions. These youngsters often report that they will "try harder," which is laudable and necessary for problem solving, but does not work if the student does not have a plan. Adolescents are often surprised to learn that motivation alone will not be effective because others' comments to them have emphasized "trying" as the primary element of success. Many adolescents with limited school success have limited patience for making plans. They engage in "one shot" thinking (Whimbey & Lockhead, 1982) and do not persist in their attempts to plan. These students need help in devising good plans before they abandon problem solving when "just trying" does not produce results. They need to learn, in their planning, to "take small bites" or to narrow the problem they are attacking and to take "baby steps," that is, to make realistic workable plans that offer a good chance of succeeding.

Schwartz and Perkins (1994) defined four levels of metacognition in problem solving. First, there is the "tacit" level in which students may be unaware of their metacognitive knowledge. That is, they may know that there is a problem, but may not be consciously reflecting on what they know. Second, there is the "awareness" level in which students may know about their metacognitive knowledge but are not acting strategically in view of this knowledge. Third, there is the "strategic" level in which students organize their thinking in problem solving, decision making, evidence seeking, and so forth. Finally, there is the "reflective" level in which students are strategic and reflective about thinking in progress, pondering and revising as needed (p. 102). In our work with adolescents, we need to help them develop through these stages of awareness and planning.

London's (1993) work in devising a curriculum of non-routine problems in math, presented a model for helping high school students become better thinkers and problem solvers. His goal was to encourage mature math thinking in adolescents and, in this effort, he regularly assigned projects requiring at least a week's work and included questions that did not have one correct answer. He wanted to discourage students' expecting to always produce quick answers. London included non-math projects to show students that problem solving underlies learning, regardless of the content. Students were required to discuss and critique each other's work in these week-long projects, presumably identifying problems and attempting to revise solutions in this process. London suggested that students need to discover, with support, that problems are often difficult, that they may not be able to think of a solution quickly and may need to tolerate ambiguity, that they may make many nonproductive attempts before solving a problem, and that they need to persist in trying a variety of approaches until the problem and solution become clear. London found that students discovered in this curriculum the necessity for noticing and examining contradictions or inaccuracies, in other words, to pay close attention and to monitor the meaning as they worked through problems. For adolescents to attain this understanding, of course, requires that they be asked to solve problems appropriate to their ability and that they be given support in their efforts to learn.

Adult collaborators need to notice when students are frustrated, and engage them in discussion of their strategies. They can encourage brainstorming with an adult or with other students at these times and/or they can model ways to proceed. Adults may facilitate successful problem solving in these cases, by presenting an easier problem or by recalling a previous problem that has been solved successfully and discussing exactly what the student did in that case. An evolving "script" for problem solving can be made explicit through this kind of guided practice (see Box 3–4). When difficulties are encountered, the student learns to persist; identifies and resolves contradictions or mistakes in problem solving attempts; accepts ambiguity as natural in problem solving; does not accept the first solution if a more effective one can be reached; and tries something instead of simply giving up when a problem seems too hard. London stressed throughout his paper, however, that one cannot simply tell students to proceed in

---

BOX 3–4: *Developing an Effective Problem Solving Script (London, 1993)*

1. Do not stop when the problem is difficult—try something else.
2. Identify and resolve contradictions or mistakes in solutions.
3. Accept ambiguity as natural when one begins to problem solve.
4. Do not automatically accept the first solution. It can lead to a better one.

---

these ways. Rather, they must experience guided problem solving to appreciate how to do it effectively.

It is helpful to demonstrate in mini-lessons various approaches to specific problems and to engage students in identifying efforts that do not include a plan at all; those with ineffective or incomplete plans as compared with good plans; to ask students to improve ineffective plans and, finally, to work together in defining and devising "good" plans. If this is a part of the thinking and proceeding in each class, students will regularly focus on problems pertinent to the discipline in question, become aware of the attributes of good plans and accumulate a repertoire of solutions matched to specific problems. It is productive to learn to problem solve while also learning needed content.

Helping Adolescents Implement Plans

Finally, there is the group of adolescents that identifies academic problems well and even makes good plans, but cannot make themselves follow through to implement the plans. Their lack of motivation, then, becomes the new problem and plans must be made to overcome this hurdle. Students have to learn within a problem solving approach that there is no quick solution or pill that can be taken to make them suddenly successful in learning or life and that the process is ongoing. The "recursive rhythm" necessary for higher-level learning has to be made clear. The importance of returning for an informed second look as a necessary expected part of the problem solving process must be demonstrated to be appreciated by adolescents. (Nelson, 1998, p. 446). Students may be more willing to work at implementing plans when they realize that identifying and making plans are strengths for them, and that mastering the last part of the problem solving process, implementing, entails the same skills.

■□ SUMMARY

A problem solving, shoulder-to-shoulder approach should address learning issues specifically and productively. In classrooms, small group or individual collaborations, students can be engaged in identifying problems within learning, in creating plans, evaluating and revising those plans, and implementing them. This process can be modeled as problems occur spontaneously or it can be taught directly through mini-lessons and applied through assignments. Posters can be displayed to remind students of the steps in problem solving in a variety of situations. It is important that problem solving be presented as an ongoing process inherent in all learning rather than just a "unit" to be covered at the beginning of a course. The IDEAL problem solver model (Bransford & Stein, 1984) includes identifying the problem, defining the problem or narrowing it to be specific, exploring alternative solutions or approaches to the problem, acting on the plan, and looking at the effects of the plan. Students need guidance in working through this cycle and returning to it when plans are not working.

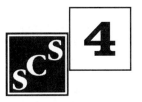

Profiles of Adolescents and Young Adults

This chapter describes adolescents who can benefit from the problem solving, shoulder-to-shoulder approach. These profiles are based on students I have known and I hope will evoke readers' experiences with similar youngsters. It is important to remember, however, that each student is an individual with unique contributions to our understanding. This should be apparent through the descriptions. Some were seen for short-term consultation, and others were engaged in lengthy collaboration, but all had something to contribute to the process. One advantage for the adult collaborator using this approach is the opportunity to learn from the adolescent and to become a better working professional with each collaboration. These profiles suggest insights provided by adolescents.

■❑ MICHAEL "I THINK I HAVE A MEMORY PROBLEM IN CLASS BUT I CAN REMEMBER FOOTBALL PLAYS."

Michael was a junior in high school and a natural athlete who played a variety of sports with ease and success. He had difficulty in history class, however, which he attributed to a "bad memory." After some discussion, Michael remarked, "You know what? I can remember the football plays better than those guys who make good grades. Isn't that funny?" With further discussion, Michael seemed to realize that his memory was not really the problem in his classroom learning. He was having trouble taking in the information in history class, that is, in listening and comprehending the myriad facts and novel concepts presented in academic-style language. He couldn't remember what he had not understood. In football, however, Michael brought extensive experience and natural proclivity to the learning experience. He understood and therefore remembered.

Diagnostic testing and prior reports established word decoding and spelling as major problem areas that interfered in Michael's reading and notetaking. A notetaker was provided and this accommodation was appropriate; however, Michael reported that he was bored in history class. His mind "drifted" he said, no matter how good his intention.

I wanted to illustrate active learning to Michael and did so by invoking his way of learning new football plays. I suggested (guessed!) that, when the coach outlined a new play on the chalkboard, Michael probably tried to guess the purpose of the play ("What is he trying to get at ... to achieve with this play?"). Michael confirmed that this was, in fact, what he would do in that situation. I went on to suggest that he probably rehearsed or walked through, in his mind, his part in the new football play, even as he sat in his seat in the coach's office. Michael agreed that this was what he did and seemed amazed that I knew these things about football, which he had not really considered a learning activity. I was able to use his natural learning to illustrate active processing, to show my delight that he was already learning in this way, and to point out how effective this was for him. He remembered those football plays because he had worked actively in learning and storing them.

I asked Michael to contrast his way of attending in this football example with what he was doing in history class. We both agreed that he was drifting because he was so inactive in this class. He needed a way to keep his mind on the discussion. He needed active listening strategies. We settled on a plan that included Michael's previewing the chapter before class. He could skip hard words and still get the "gist" of the chapter by reading the title, looking at the pictures and reading the summary. This would give him information to guide his listening. He might be less overloaded with new information and more able to listen during discussion if he came into class with this "warm up" (see Chapter 7). The second active listening strategy Michael agreed to try was writing key words (or even just the first letter of a word when spelling was a problem). He could then compare his key words with those of his notetaker to see if he was identifying important facts in this shorthand way. Michael practiced these strategies and later proved that he had really appreciated the concept of active listening.

Because of Michael's extreme decoding problems, I suggested that he be given recorded textbooks and he was amenable to the idea. This was my first experience with recorded texts and I assumed, naively, that it would be a simple solution—just plug Michael in and let him learn! Michael returned after the first week with this comment, "Dr. Tattershall, I need some active listening strategies for these tapes. I drift just like I do in class." Michael was the more effective partner at this phase of the collaboration because he had clearly identified his problem and I learned a lesson. Of course he drifted when listening to the recorded text. These were the same unfamiliar topics and difficult language he was having trouble with in class. So we practiced previewing the chapter as he had been doing for class and for the same reason—to develop background information, a context for the specific learning. After the previewing, Michael was guided in listening to the chapter a section at a time, making key word notes after each section. Michael had discovered his problem in listening, had adopted the appropriate goal of active listening, had generalized it to a new situation and learned specific strategies for implementing this goal. This was an effective collaboration.

■ TYREL "NOBODY HAS TO TAKE SHOP, BUT I HAVE TO TAKE ENGLISH."

Tyrel was a graduating senior who was especially talented in woodworking skills. His shop teacher had never had a student with the natural abilities that Tyrel showed early in the semester and felt he was destined to craft fine furniture. Tyrel was frustrated, however, that "Nobody has to take shop so they don't see how good I am, but I have to take English." His learning problems showed up where language skills were required and, because his spelling was a problem, he made it a practice to use only simple words in his writing assignments. This began to bother him in his senior year, however, because he felt that he had a good vocabulary that he was not using in his writing. He decided to write an assigned paper and to let his natural vocabulary flow in the rough draft without worrying about spelling. His brother then proofread it for him, which seemed like a good plan, but it backfired. Tyrel's English teacher had become accustomed to his use of common words that he could spell and, presumably, the simple language consistent with those words. She did not recognize the higher-level writing he produced in his last paper and accused him of having had someone else write his paper. Tyrel was furious.

We were able to discuss this episode and Tyrel seemed to appreciate that the teacher's reaction was to be expected because he had been writing in a limited way throughout the year. It was tempting to dwell on how sad it was that he had not thought of this brother-as-proofreader plan early in his high school career, but that would have been unproductive. It seemed more appropriate to stress the good problem solving that Tyrel had applied to get past the spelling problem and use his vocabulary knowledge in his writing, finally, of this last paper. He had spent time and energy to figure out a way to write using his own vocabulary. To capitalize on this experience, it would have been appropriate to design a "blitz" writing plan to make up for lost writing time and to allow Tyrel to exercise his higher level language skills. We could have analyzed his spelling together to see how many spellings would be identified and corrected by a spell checker that might be more available than his brother. Tyrel was not patient enough to embark on an extensive spelling remediation program but he was amenable to setting an initial goal of achieving phonetically close spellings so that he could better utilize a spell check. Giving a student shared ownership for planning means that they do not always choose to work on everything we recommend. Tyrel's solution seemed reasonable.

■□ MACK "LET'S TALK ABOUT WORLD WAR II. I HAVE TROUBLE PAYING ATTENTION TO THE BORING STUFF."

Mack was observed in a variety of situations waiting in an anteroom, working within individual intervention sessions, and participating in a small group class. Although he was always polite, Mack often seemed lethargic, to lack active interest in ongoing learning activities. He had been delayed in his early language development and retained a somewhat stilted speech pattern, suggesting persistent verbal apraxia. His language was adequate for short conversational exchanges; however, Mack had always been slow in finishing written work in class and needed close supervision in his homework. This picture changed when Mack was talking, reading or writing about his favorite subjects World War II, the Korean War, Vietnam and current events. Mack was an expert on these subjects and pursued information avidly. He could discuss these topics effectively and took every opportunity to learn more about them. There seemed to be no middle ground for Mack—either his great interest kept him active or he returned to his pleasant but passive self, a disadvantage when he was studying topics outside of his passionate interest.

Mack did not seem aware of this attention style and seemed like other students who have volunteered that they are unable to pay attention to "the boring stuff." However, he seemed clearly to be in that group who need extraordinary interest in order to maintain ordinary attention. Levine (1990) described this attention style that seems to reflect an arousal system clearly dependent on high interest. I recognized it in Mack and others. Mack's mother quit her job to supervise his homework throughout his high school years. Hers was a difficult task—to allow Mack time for current events, that he loved, but to help him also reserve time for other assignments that were much less interesting to him.

Mack was seen for an in-depth evaluation of his learning problems after his senior year in high school and the neuropsychologist assured his parents that Mack had been doing the best he could in his approach to studying. These parents, in desperation, had held out prizes most teenagers would have worked hard for, but Mack did not respond with extended effort. The neurologist said that their attempts to motivate Mack were admirable but could not have worked given his very real attention problems. Medication was prescribed to aid Mack in his attention during his first year in college. Mack was apparently included in the discussion of medication, but opted to try college without medication and, in his first semester, attended only the classes that interested him. It appeared that Mack may not have clearly understood his attention style and the need for help from medication and/or may just not have agreed with the finding. In any case, his very problem, lethargy in attention outside his areas of interest, may have worked against his being an active collaborator in his own problem solving. In this case, the shoulder-to-shoulder approach would have required frequent and ongoing clarification of Mack's understanding of the conclusions of others and how they arrived at those conclusions. It would be important to ensure that Mack contributed his own opinions about problems and plans as he tended to be so passive. His mother had been vigilant in keeping him on the tasks necessary for school, but Mack may not have understood what she was doing and why it was necessary. Without being involved actively in problem solving, it is unlikely that Mack would notice ongoing problems; know that he should make plans and/or monitor the effect of the plans. Students like Mack, who attend actively within their passionate interests but not in other contexts, often are misjudged by teachers who assume that, because they can pursue some topics avidly, they are just not trying in other instances ("Come on, Mack. How can you know so much about WW II and not know these formulas?"). These teachers and the students themselves often do not realize that adolescents like Mack require *extraordinary* interest to maintain *ordinary* attention to a task, an observation that needs to be discovered, understood by all involved and to become the focus for planning. Mack and others with the same attention style might need to study in a room near others, for instance, so they don't drift away to their favorite topics. They may need to read aloud to keep their interest or even to stand up as they read. A variety of plans could be generated followed by guided practice, evaluation and revision. In any case, with this attention style, a conscious plan is necessary for maintaining attention to the "boring stuff."

The student needs to understand the plan, agree to it, have help in establishing a habit of using the plan and be guided in evaluating and revising the plan periodically as needed.

■ SALLY "I HAVE THIS PAPER TO WRITE AND I DON'T KNOW WHERE TO START."

Sally, a high school senior, announced that she had a paper to write for school but had not yet started; that she always had trouble thinking of writing topics and in getting started on a writing assignment. After finding out what was allowable in this assignment, I asked Sally which topic she found interesting and she chose "hobbies." I suggested she list all the hobbies that came to mind, and sports dominated her list.

She chose softball and, again on request, listed words that came to mind when she thought of this topic. She then grouped her brainstormed words into apparent categories and, on request, wrote a sentence about each group of words. We discussed the ideas to provoke further thinking about what she might write about softball given these prewriting, brainstorming activities.

It seemed clear from her comments that Sally was going to write an informative paper for a naive reader, one who knew very little about softball. I then asked Sally to look over her list, categories and sentences before engaging in a timed writing exercise, that is, nonstop writing for one minute intervals. After three minutes, Sally read aloud from what she had written.

The first line she read was quite surprising: "Softball is a loving sport." I was intrigued by "loving" and asked her what she meant by that statement. She explained that she had played softball with the same group of girls for many years and the friendships were so important to her that she couldn't imagine playing with another team. She had found her main idea and it was very different from what I had expected. What had seemed a rather dry informative piece about the game of softball, became an explanation of the relationships among her teammates. Sally had a good start, then, on her paper and it would definitely be *her* idea, her feelings and her voice.

This was a clear example of how collaboration can work. As the professional, I provided the structure of the lesson and Sally provided her unique perspective on the topic. Her voice appeared within the process I had directed. Shoulder-to-shoulder we had each contributed to this particular writing experience.

◼◻ SHEILA " OH, I'M SORRY. COULDN'T YOU HEAR ME?"

Sheila was standing in the waiting room with her mother as I approached. We exchanged smiles and introductions, an unremarkable event to casual observers, but I could feel my brow begin to wrinkle and questions coming to mind. "Doesn't she seem young for a senior in high school? Why? She's standing too close to her mother, perhaps for her culture and age. She's smiling nicely but didn't she look down a little rather than straight at me when we introduced ourselves? "

Our work had begun. Sheila was already providing information, albeit unconsciously, and I was mulling it over. Sheila was average in height, a little taller than I, but when she sat down she seemed to shrink, to fold into herself. With her arms held tightly to her body, she slumped a little, tilted her head down toward her chest, and glanced at me out of the corner of her eye. When she talked, she mumbled, using very little lip movement, although there were no specific misarticulations in her speech. She answered questions with short answers, smiled appropriately at humorous remarks but initiated few comments of her own. She exuded poor self-esteem, or shyness, or both.

In the midst of our lackluster interchange, however, something interesting happened. Sheila raised her chin to look directly at me and the effect was startling. She looked very different. Holding her chin up showed off her best features, her oval face and graceful neck. This made her look more bold and her voice easier to hear. It was clear that Sheila needed to increase her use of direct eye contact and to speak in a louder voice in order to achieve a more assertive communication effect. Sheila had now provided a good way to begin.

I suggested an assignment requiring Sheila to use this "chin up" posture in certain situations that week. With her assent, her mother was involved in noting and counting instances when Sheila's chin was up at unassigned times during the week. I asked Sheila to explain her understanding of the assignment and the reasons for it. I wanted to be sure that she understood my intent. Then, I asked if this assignment seemed appropriate and reasonable. Sheila seemed to feel that it was and she was interested. The first session had gone well. Specific problem areas and goals seemed clear and Sheila had provided a way to begin working on them. We had made a good start on our joint venture.

■ TIM "WHY HASN'T ANYONE EVER TOLD ME THIS BEFORE?"

Tim seemed self-assured as he talked and joked freely in a study strategies class for college bound students. He had just completed his senior year in high school and, by his own admission, had cheated through much of his school career. He had been a successful athlete and had recently received a football scholarship to a religious college. He seemed eager to turn over a new leaf in his life and change his "cheating ways" by learning other strategies for academic survival.

Tim was very attentive to the class activities and subsequent discussion about studying. He seemed amazed that, just as in sports, there were specific, known strategies one could learn and apply in schoolwork. One day he could contain himself no longer and he blurted out, "Why hasn't anyone ever told me all this before?" His tone suggested that people had conspired to withhold school learning strategies from him, that this was good "stuff" and he should have known about it before.

Tim made a good point. He needed to be taught how to study. He had figured out ways to cheat on his own but he needed help in acquiring legitimate strategies. His comment echoed the sentiment of a teacher who was introduced in the early 1980s to language learning issues in early literacy with implications for teaching and she also asked accusingly, "Why haven't I been told about this before?"

Both teachers and students need specific discussion of ways to process information in learning. Tim had assumed as do so many students without natural school learning talent that learning equals already knowing; that there are the "haves" (the ones who automatically have answers) and the "have-nots" (the ones like me). Many adolescents with learning problems do not appreciate that learning *is* problem solving; that it is not always a *have* versus *have-not* proposition, and that any learner will have to problem solve at some point, no matter how automatic their learning seems. Tim was a practical learner who would naturally problem solve outside of school, but he had not realized that the process was similar in school; that one identifies the problem specifically, makes a plan and implements it. Unfortunately, the class that Tim attended was an introduction to many strategies without the long-term collaboration that would have allowed Tim to identify his own problems as they occurred within his own curriculum. He liked the idea of being given solutions, but like the short-lived storage of isolated facts mentioned by the comedian cited in Chapter 1, strategies taught aside from Tim's real problems might also be lost after a short time. One cannot just "tell" problem solving—it must be shown through ongoing joint collaboration. Perhaps, a college tutor guided him through further development as a learner.

■□ LISA "WHEN I HEARD THOSE FOREIGN NAMES, I STOPPED LISTENING."

Lisa was included in a small group exercise (Main Idea Evolving) in which the instructor lectured about the life of a Haitian poet. The students were asked to listen and to recall facts that were then listed on the chalkboard. They listened to the short lecture for a second time and were asked to add to or to correct their list of recalled facts and then to decide upon the most important ideas. Lisa contributed very few comments until the instructor asked, in the spirit of the problem solving approach, for the group to reflect on the experience, "What was hard about this exercise? What did you do when you had a problem?" Lisa was the first to report that "When I heard those foreign names, I just stopped listening because I knew I wouldn't understand anything after that."

With further discussion, it seemed clear that Lisa felt she had to be sure of everything as she listened or subsequent information would be too difficult to understand. Her reading comprehension strategies were different, however, because she could suspend her concern when she encountered new words or concepts in reading and skip the unknown word to use subsequent context to uncover its meaning. In listening she became quickly frustrated if she did not understand everything as it occurred because she couldn't skip a word and come back to it.

Although Lisa had a clear understanding of her problem in listening, she did not have an effective solution. Hers was an all-or-none approach to a listening task, and she seemed to regularly react in this way. She seemed to assume that there was no solution possible; that she came into this world with this stigma and it could not be overcome.

Lisa's becoming overloaded with new information in listening is a problem encountered by many students, particularly in social studies and science classes where there is often a heavy dose of new information to process. Lisa and other students with this style should be introduced to a variety of ways to "warm up" to a topic beforehand in order to lighten the information processing load in class. If Lisa had been introduced first to the overall facts of this Haitian poet's life, the specific vocabulary might not have been as important for processing.

Lisa's listening problems were complicated by allergies that sometimes caused a fluctuation in hearing over a month's time, from excellent to a severe bilateral loss. Unlike her frustration with new information, which she had clearly identified as a listening problem, Lisa was unaware of her hearing problems. One day, she seemed particularly visually attentive, and I asked if she were having difficulty hearing me. She said "No, I don't think so," but continued to look closely at me as a I spoke. A hearing screening that day showed a severe bilateral loss (70 dB threshold across the audiogram for both ears). Subsequent weekly screenings showed steady improvement with excellent hearing levels by the end of a month. Because of the fluctuating and gradual nature of her periods of hearing loss, Lisa apparently had adjusted her visual attention as needed without awareness of her hearing problems. One wonders if this had occurred throughout Lisa's life during allergy season, and how it had contributed to her listening style and learning problems. Lisa was treated for allergies and began to monitor her hearing more consciously. Lisa and I were unable to work extensively on prelistening "warm-up" strategies, but they would have been helpful for listening and reading in class and for more effective speechreading in conversations during allergy periods.

Lisa had reading decoding problems as well, and came into one therapy session with the announcement "Oh, Dr. Tattershall, when I read I never know whether a word says "has" or "was," and I am so afraid I'll mess up on one of these words ." Again, Lisa had identified a problem accurately, but seemed not to know a solution. In an effort to clearly define the problem, I asked her to read aloud and we discovered that she always read "was" correctly but overgeneralized this word to include the word "has" which she usually read as "was." The opposite ("has" for "was") did not occur. It was apparent in trial practice, that Lisa needed to and could use sentence context and first letter to identify "has."

I discussed this "was-has" issue with Lisa in order to make these points: 1) she had identified a specific problem herself; 2) we needed to study the problem in order to further understand it; 3) knowing that she read the word "was" correctly but also used it for "has" suggested a clear plan—be vigilant for these words in print and when one of them is encountered, look closely at the first letter; and 4) she would have to consciously practice using this strategy to correct the problem. This seems so simple but provided an opportunity to clearly understand the way Lisa proceeded. She typically stopped after identifying problems and became emotional about her difficulty, which prevented more effective problem solving. Lisa needed to know what she was doing and to have a better approach to problem solving, to stop at these times, identify the problem, make a plan, then try it out. She also needed supportive guidance in establishing this approach.

Lisa entered our office on another occasion with this statement, "I feel so dumb. I cannot even read this magazine!" She may have been correct about her struggle with reading in this case, but I was struck with her quick assumption that her learning inadequacies were always the one and only cause of difficulty. She seemed unaware that the magazine article could have been poorly written, for instance. This tunnel vision is one of the serious side effects of having a diagnostic label. Adolescents who have struggled with various learning difficulties often assume that every problem is caused to their label—learning or reading problems, attention deficit, language disorders, and so forth. They are correct that many problems they encounter, particularly in learning, do reflect their identified diagnoses, but not all. Regardless of the cause, however, problems need to be solved. These youngsters, including Lisa, need help in looking beyond their own limitations to solutions. They need to appreciate through a collaborative approach that problem solving is what everyone does and so must they; that their learning problems may be severe making problem solving more critical for success, but that identifying and solving problems is an effective, necessary process for everyone. This point is made not by telling students but by showing through problem solving focused on their own needs within a supportive relationship.

■□ JUAN "NO, I'M NOT HAVING ANY TROUBLE PAYING ATTENTION."

Juan had suffered a head injury in an auto accident on a trip home from college and he had been seen for language therapy by several clinicians within a one-on-one approach. His attention was adequate within individual conversations, but he presented differently in a group setting. In a class for young adults with head injury problems, Juan often seemed to drift in his attention and to be unaware of doing so. When asked if he were having "trouble staying with us, staying attentive?" he said that he did not think so.

It was interesting, however, that on two occasions Juan came into the class very energized. Once he was excited about an old friend coming into town and, on the second occasion, he was thrilled at having recovered his long-lost class ring. These happy events seemed to buoy Juan's spirits and the increased emotion seemed to help him sustain attention throughout these two class sessions. In terms of conscious monitoring, however, Juan did not seem to notice when his attention was waning, so he did not think to problem solve on his own. Had we continued with the collaboration, videotapes might have helped Juan become aware of his variable attention. Family members could have alerted him to his drifting attention and perhaps identified times of day or situations in which he was more or less alert. In any case, it would have been difficult to make plans to solve Juan's attention problems until he clearly identified the problem.

■❏ JAN "YES, UH HUH, OH … I HAVE NO IDEA WHAT YOU SAID."

Jan was a stunning teenager with extraordinary musical talents and fashion taste to match but she had a sad educational history that included attendance at a variety of schools without success. She was so attractive and personable that her learning problems may have been masked in school.

Within a consultation session to help Jan develop better comprehension abilities, she appeared to be listening attentively to an explanation. She maintained good eye contact and nodded appropriately as though she were following the ideas being presented. At an appropriate stopping place, I said, "Jan, I want to see if I am making sense here. Tell me, in your own words, what you think I have said about this topic." Jan paused but could not recall and/or explain anything that had been said. Both she and I were surprised because she had responded nonverbally as though she were actively processing my explanation.

One wonders if Jan's musical ability has helped her attend to the rhythm of conversation and to pause appropriately without really listening to the content. She may go on "automatic pilot" while listening much like parents do at the end of the day when children are chattering away. Parents may know that they are not actively attending but until this particular comprehension check, Jan did not realize that she could look and feel as though she were listening and, yet, not be taking in information at all. One wonders if her talent in backchanneling contributed to her learning problems not being identified. Jan was instrumental in teaching me always to check understanding by asking for a paraphrase, rather than assuming understanding from nonverbal feedback. It was always clear when Juan's attention faded because he did not look like he was listening, but Jan seemed very engaged. Like Juan, though, she was unaware of her listening problem and needed help in starting the problem solving process by becoming acutely aware of when, where, and under what specific conditions her listening problems occurred. Jan needed help in noticing when she "fazed out" and to practice checking her listening by periodically stopping the speaker and restating what she thought the person had said. In a classroom situation, Jan would need to be an expert on the usual class routine, the instructor's signals for attention and transitions, and to regularly restate oral directions or explanations of concepts to ensure active processing.

MARIA "OH YES, I WANT TO BE A TEACHER."

Maria was tested within a program to identify transition needs of high school seniors with a history of learning problems. Her scores showed extremely low academic skills and limited interest in academic subjects so her stated interest in becoming a teacher was surprising. She seemed to know little about what was required in order to become a teacher and/or if this goal was appropriate for her. She was typical of many youngsters who seem to know little about themselves as learners even after having had special placement in school, individual educational plans, and diagnostic testing completed every three years. The learning interview is particularly helpful in identifying students' knowledge about their own learning and/or world knowledge pertinent to transitions to work or extended learning. Early collaboration seems extremely important to prevent this disparity between ability, interest and intentions. Maria should have been drawn into academic planning earlier so she could be more realistic in setting goals and/or could appreciate the work that would be required to achieve her goals.

It is possible that Maria could, if motivated, guided and given appropriate accommodations, develop skills commensurate with her goals. The important issue in this collaboration, it seemed, was for the adult to help Maria make her own informed decision and not to discourage her prematurely. With information and motivation, she might outstrip the adult's expectations but hers needs to be an informed plan with self-awareness and knowledge of what is entailed in reaching her goals.

BERT "OH YES, I ALWAYS DO ALL THAT AND MORE WHEN I STUDY."

Bert was given a battery of learning style and strategy assessments. His responses suggested that he was a model of active learning. He seemed to know what he was *supposed* to do as a student, but not to be aware of what he was *actually* doing. Although he could decode words very well, he didn't attend well to his reading, so his mother regularly read homework reading assignments to him. I asked her to videotape a homework session because I wanted to see Bert in action. In this taped homework session, his mother read a paragraph and asked him if there were any new terms that he did not understand. He replied that there were none. Then, because his mother knew Bert well, she selected several words to check his understanding and he was unable to explain the meaning of any of these words. Bert didn't seem to appreciate the disparity between his reported and his actual study habits. He typically showed a very concrete and direct language style, so I assumed that he was not trying to "con" me. He was doing well in school because he was being given excellent help both at school and at home. Unfortunately, as a high school junior, he was not actively engaged in his own learning. Others were accommodating in ways that he did not realize, and others were helping in ways that he had not taken as his own strategies. So, with his senior year looming and college after that, this young man had been taken through his own curriculum without learning much about learning.

A major goal was for Bert to become more active in and knowledgeable about his own learning, that is, to identify specific strategies his mother used during various study tasks and to adopt them himself when he could. He also needed to know what accommodations teachers were making for him, the reasons why these accommodations were appropriate for him, and how to advocate for similar accommodations on his own. After he knew what others were doing to help, Bert would have to practice using those strategies throughout his senior year in preparation for college. He would, we hope, know what to do on his own and what to ask for in accommodations for learning.

■□ SEAN "I DIDN'T WANT TO COME TO THIS CLASS. MY MOM MADE ME."

Sean was enrolled in a study strategies class designed to teach middle and high school students specific ways to approach their school work. This class encouraged students to notice classroom routines and teacher signals for initial attention or for a change in activities, to develop specific plans for organizing schoolwork and materials; and to find active ways to process information in study, among other issues. Sean's class was one of four small groups meeting in different classrooms. The instructors rotated among the classes to allow observations of different teacher styles and I taught Sean's class on the second day of the series.

Sean pulled his chair away from the group and was sitting by the window, clearly separated from the class activity. He volunteered few comments and seemed to indicate with his body language that he was not going to be a part of this class. When I asked him directly how he studied, Sean said that he usually sat on the couch, turned the lights down low and wrapped himself in a blanket before beginning his homework, a routine that suggested he had no intention of working hard at homework—no matter what we said in this class. As the instructor that day, I wanted to focus on organization for study, that is, making good systems for managing homework problems. I also wanted to find a way to draw Sean into the group.

I asked Sean what he liked to do in his free time and he grudgingly reported that he worked on the family cars. I asked how they stored their tools in his family, if they hung the tools on pegboards, used a tool box or what? Sean said they kept their tools in drawers. I asked if they put all the tools together in a drawer or if they separated them and he explained how they put different types of tools in different drawers. He turned toward the group and spoke somewhat louder as he explained the way his tools were kept and he seemed to enter the discussion in spite of himself. I pointed out that his seemed like a good way to keep track of tools and to have them available when needed—a good system.

This tool storing system provided the real world example for the premise of the lesson, that is, that successful students devise or learn systematic ways to solve organizational problems. Sean looked somewhat surprised that he had not only been engaged in the discussion, but that his was a central role. Sean was clearly one who had never appreciated the relationship between what he did at home and what one should do in school. He was like others who seem to proceed well as problem solvers outside of school. They are not discouraged when one idea does not work, will persist in trying other ideas, can often work in poor conditions without proper materials and still be able to create something effective. These same students seem to abandon good thinking at school, assuming that their kind of thinking does not apply there; that school information and tasks are so totally different from real world experience that out-of-school logic does not apply. Sean was a reluctant collaborator in this interchange, but his willingness to share his experience was encouraging. Given enough opportunities to see that he had information and skills of value in, and not separate from, school learning, Sean might soften his resistance, become an effective collaborator and improve his learning.

■◻ PAUL "DID YOU SAY I MISSED A COUPLE OF WORDS? REALLY? WHATEVER YOU SAY."

Paul was a very cooperative thirteen year old who seemed motivated to do well and even asked for homework in our sessions. He complied with every request and seemed to enjoy a challenge, but initiated little and seemed to have difficulty in sustained listening. He always knew the gist of the subject but did not attend to specific detail in listening or reading.

Paul's mother brought him for evaluation in order to plan a more effective home schooling program. She expressed concern that Paul did not seem to know much about his own learning; that he often "has the skill but has not yet mastered the concept" in many lessons. She said that Paul enjoyed hands-on projects and investigations but did not generalize what he learned to new situations.

It seemed important that Paul become aware of his passive style in listening and reading. Because he usually understood the overall idea, he seemed not to appreciate the need to attend to detail. He was not identifying this problem, and yet I saw this as an important issue. This was a dilemma in our collaboration—Paul and I did not have a shared focus. He was unaware of his tendency to neglect detail. My tack was to engage Paul in oral reading followed by "proof-listening." In this activity, Paul read aloud into a tape recorder and I wrote his miscues on my copy of his reading passage. He was then asked to listen to his oral reading while visually reviewing the text and to mark any inaccuracies in his oral reading of the material. We then compared his proofing with my copy and recorded his rate of accuracy in identifying miscues through proof-listening. Paul was then asked to reread the material, to "proof-listen" again and he always increased his reading accuracy on the second trial.

I checked Paul's understanding of what we had done in every session (and why) and asked his opinion of what we were doing. Rather than trying to convince him through discussion or argument that he had a problem in attention, I wanted to discover, along with him, exactly what his attention patterns were and how they changed over time.

Paul presented a special challenge to the shoulder-to-shoulder approach because he was so compliant. It was easy to take the lead because he would follow amiably, without active attention or understanding in the initial sessions. I had to consciously plan for Paul to make more decisions and take a more active part in our sessions. The box metaphor came back to haunt me. As the adult in charge of setting the outer limits of the lessons, I seemed to be making the box too small. Paul's part in the process was limited and passive. Using the transactional model, the arrows were all starting with me going toward Paul and coming back. I had to change our collaboration so that I did less and Paul did more. It was important to enhance Paul's awareness of his attention problems and for him to check his understanding of what we were doing; but it was critical that he also be involved in identifying specific problems, making plans and evaluating. Boxes and arrows helped me consider and reconsider Paul's part in our collaboration. Paul was younger than Bert and I wanted him to avoid being pushed along by adults in order to succeed in school without his really being involved.

■ SUSAN "RECORDED TEXTBOOKS? NO, I'VE NEVER HEARD OF THOSE. MATH IS EASY FOR ME."

Susan was a high school junior with reading at the third grade level and spelling at fourth grade level. She had opted out of special classes because she felt that the "other kids needed it more, and I really wasn't getting any help." She was in all regular classes without any accommodations. She said that all but one of her classes required daily textbook reading and she sometimes had to read orally in class, which she hated. She said that she had particular difficulty in history because of the amount of new information to be learned. She said that her spelling was bad, but she had no other difficulty in writing. Susan responded thoughtfully to all questions within the learning interview and seemed to have a good idea of her strengths and weaknesses. She seemed very troubled by history class and mentioned it several times. She was quiet and didn't initiate many other comments so I was surprised when she reported that she asked questions freely in class. I wondered if she really did.

I only saw Susan once but I had heard her story before—a youngster who had appropriate social skills but could not participate fully in classes because of learning problems. I couldn't imagine how she managed reading assignments and taking notes without accommodations. I wondered why she hadn't collaborated with anyone to make a good plan that included protection from oral reading without prior notice. This is one of the important questions on the learning interview ("How do you feel about reading orally in class? What classes require this?), and it often leads to an immediate effort to protect students from having to read orally. Teachers often have students read orally in class to ensure that they will, in fact, read the material. They also call on students randomly apparently to keep them vigilant in their listening. This pressure can be very unfair to the poor reader.

Before I reflected on Susan's test results in general, I suggested that she arrange with her teacher to volunteer to read aloud in class, rather than being called on unexpectedly, so she could practice a particular passage ahead of time each day. She seemed willing and unafraid to explain to her teacher that she had difficulty reading and to appreciate that this plan would allow her to read more effectively in class. Although Susan did not seem assertive, she explained that in her small school everyone knew that she had learning problems so asking for this accommodation would not be a risky thing to do.

The next pressing need for Susan was to obtain recorded textbooks, but with the understanding that she have someone guide her in learning to use them and that the helper stay with her until she was comfortable with this tool. Her reading comprehension was a relative strength compared with her poor word decoding, and she did not seem to have a "short fuse" for struggle. This profile, in my experience, made her a very good candidate for using recorded textbooks. She may also have been willing to tape record class lectures and discussions. Many high school students are hesitant to tape record because this draws attention to them in class, so teachers will sometimes take responsibility for the tape recorder. Susan might have felt comfortable recording the lecture in history class where she had difficulty with the excessive amount of information. She would have to continue trying to take some notes in class to make it easier to "fill in" information when she listened to the tape and to help her maintain active listening.

Susan impressed me as mature and reflective for her age. With the appropriate accommodations and guidance in using and practicing them in her remaining time in high school, Susan seemed a good candidate for attending junior college, a hope she expressed.

■□ STACI "NO, I DON'T KNOW WHAT TO WRITE DOWN. I TRY TO LEARN EVERYTHING!"

Staci had been an average student in high school; very social; a cheerleader with supportive, interested parents who provided all the amenities of higher middle class . She went off to college with high hopes and worked hard by all accounts, but had failing grades at the end of the first semester. She had recently undergone a complete educational evaluation and was referred to our center for intervention. Staci and her family were seen for an initial consultation to review their understanding of her evaluation results and to allow them to add their own observations to the formal test findings. This discussion was extremely helpful in making the formal testing results meaningful.

Staci's father commented that he thought his daughter had not applied herself and was "partying too much" in her first year in college. When he looked over her notes for one of the classes she had failed, however, he was amazed at the extensive effort she had apparently put into her notes. As he put it, "You could have published those notes. They were that complete." My diagnostic antennae were activated by the word "complete" and I asked "How complete, Staci? Do you know what to write down?" She replied, "No, my friends tell me I try to write everything!" She was apparently having difficulty differentiating "wheat" from "chaff" in her notetaking (see Chapter 7).

Staci and I embarked on a short series of sessions to help her develop strategies for returning to college under the pressure of academic probation. She seemed to appreciate the need for a better plan. I assumed that a good place to start would be learning how to read a chapter using a modification of SQ3R Survey, Read, Recite, Review (Stauffer, 1969). There was no indication of language problems in Staci's evaluation report and she certainly expressed herself well within the whole family discussion, so I thought she simply needed a more organized way to study. Staci easily learned the strategy for surveying a chapter, but when she began to read within each section she clearly had difficulty understanding the complex sentences in her college text. This academic language stressed Staci's abilities in ways that conversation did not. After further discussion with Staci and her parents, however, it seemed that she did have some difficulty even within conversation. She often did not understand jokes, for instance, and simply smiled her way through many situations.

We began to attack textbook sentences with a sentence decombining exercise designed to find and highlight individual thoughts within complicated, formal sentences. Staci listened and watched as I read a sentence "Walter Cannon (1942), a well-known physiologist, studied many voodoo deaths and concluded that they are explained by changes in the body that accompany strong emotion," p. 327 (Coon, 1992). Staci was able to identify the topic stating, "This is about a well known physiologist, Walter Cannon." I then restated this sentence in statements of one thought each "Walter Cannon was a well-known physiologist. He studied many voodoo deaths. He made a conclusion. There are changes in the body. These changes accompany strong emotion. This explains the deaths." Staci began to take her turns at decombining sentences in this way and gradually to appreciate that there were individual thoughts she could find and understand within the long, complex sentences. Soon she could restate the individual thoughts relatively quickly, but when she tried to reassemble them to reconstruct the original sentence, she was unsure of how to reconnect the thoughts. At that point, she needed help in focusing on and learning to appreciate connector words for their functions in separating and connecting thoughts in particular ways. Staci learned about connectives when immersed in language that directed her attention to the connectives and discussed their use in a text, a combination of direct teaching and contextual abstraction.

The sentence decombining and recombining highlighted the individual thoughts and their connectors. It was interesting that Staci's oral reading of this material changed at this point. She had read a passage at the beginning of our work and was quite fluent, too fluent. She was reading high level expository material at the rate appropriate for a romance novel! There were no telltale pauses to show the active thinking required by college textbooks. She was apparently reading but not really processing the information. After engaging in sentence combining for several weeks, however, Staci read this kind of material with pauses that showed attention to the thoughts within sentences. She was decombining as she read. This was especially interesting because we had not discussed her original reading in terms of rate or phrasing. These surface features had improved as a result of deeper processing.

Staci seemed relieved to have a conscious strategy for reading and understanding her textbooks, but her "bag of tricks" for comprehension of higher level language was still relatively small. Serendipity was definitely at work for Staci. We located a doctoral student at Staci's college who had recently set up a successful college study strategies program in another state, and was willing to work with Staci. Staci would be able to continue her collaboration to find and practice effective studying strategies. That was my last contact with Staci, but I will be forever grateful to her for reminding me to look closely at sentence level processing in textbooks even when conversation seems to be going well and there is no prior evidence of language difficulty.

■□ SUMMARY

These youngsters represent a variety of student types. They are different from each other but there are themes that seem to run through these vignettes. Adolescents often find school topics irrelevant to their lives. Some can proceed adequately in spite of the apparent irrelevance, but others have difficulty and need help. Adolescents sometimes have practical skills that can be helpful in school, but don't realize that these approaches apply to academics. Adolescents can be unaware, specifically, of their strengths and weaknesses as learners, even when they have been tested and retested, analyzed, labeled, and given excellent help at home and in school. They cannot be their own advocates with limited self-knowledge. Adolescents often see learning as a gift that others seem to have and they lack; so when success in learning is not automatic, they give up and rarely develop a range of learning strategies because it seems futile. We have to change this picture within collaborative, shoulder-to-shoulder ongoing problem solving focused on language processing within school learning. We have to help adolescents identify problems and learn strategies for solving those problems including asking for appropriate accommodations from others.

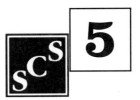

Getting to Know Adolescents: Story Swapping, Interviews and Questionnaires

In the effort to elicit information about adolescents' language and learning, informal tools can be helpful. This chapter discusses Story Swapping, the Learning Interview, the Single Class Mini-interview, the Homework Script Questionnaire, and the LASSI-HS, tools designed to elicit information directly from the adolescent client. The Parents' Observations about Language and Learning (POLL) also can provide impressions of parents who have observed their children's learning process in daily homework. The Homework Script Questionnaire can be used both with parents and students to pinpoint problems within homework. Error pattern analysis of students' own classwork, including answers to study guide papers, rough drafts of writing assignments, various kinds of tests, in-class assignments as compared with at-home work, and reading of classroom texts allows for personalized assessment pertinent to each student's experience.

■□ STORY SWAPPING

Donald Graves (1985) explained that he began every college class with story swapping, even his research design classes. He simply started every new class by telling a personal anecdote, pausing to let someone else contribute a story or by continuing to tell stories himself. His initial aim, as he explained, was to create a supportive community of learners, one in which people began to know each other as people before the formal lessons started. He wanted to know the students; to cause them to know him and each other early in the class.

If one views diagnostic measures as "getting to know you," then this is a viable activity, particularly in a group. Initially it is awkward to stand in front of a new class, particularly one filled with adolescents, and begin to tell stories. Unlike the naturalness of talking in a casual conversation, instructors' telling of stories in front of the class can seem contrived, abrupt, and certainly unexpected in a first meeting. After several anecdotes, however, there is usually a stirring in the group from those who are reminded of similar incidents in their own lives or in those of someone they know and students begin sharing stories.

Sample Stories

I have found it helpful in initiating story swapping to describe my high school band director who was greatly admired for his collection of personally autographed pictures of famous musicians he had met while playing in local bands. He continued to play at various places in our area after he retired from his high school position, and, unfortunately, was playing at a local night spot, Beverly Hills, when their cabaret room caught on fire. The exits were blocked and many people died in this fire. My band director was able to get out safely, but then returned to help others, which proved fatal for him. I usually pause and then tell about a colleague who was attending a smaller party in the front part of that same building that evening. When the fire was discovered, a waiter asked my friend and her group to exit. She said that she did not consider the fire to be serious and assumed they would be able to return quickly. She was surprised to encounter a great deal of smoke in the area near the front entrance but all their party safely exited the building and went home unaware that 152 people had died in the back of the building where the fire had started. My friend was shaken by how close she had come to being included in that group. I pause then to look for possible stories coming to mind and continue with another story if no "stirrings" seem to be evident in facial expressions or body language.

A third personal story I tell involves a strange call I received from someone posing as a policemen who had arrested a man for making obscene calls. This man, so the caller explained, had a list of women's names and my name was on the list. This caller eventually revealed himself as an impostor, but the story is interesting and amusing in contrast to the more serious fire account. There are also several accounts of auto accidents, embarrassing dating incidents and pet adventures that have been productive in eliciting stories from others.

After listening for awhile, students in the group begin to offer their own stories. The atmosphere changes to that of casual conversations where one story leads to another and their stories introduce people in memorable ways. Groups form more quickly than with the typical routine in which people simply state their names, where they live, and so forth. In one class, for instance, a young woman told us about an incident that had involved her sister, and in telling this story also informed us about what this sister was like, how she was different from another sibling, and what the family typically expected from each of these girls. The young woman who was telling this story provided a good language sample that showed her communication style and ability to relate a narrative. I can still visualize this storyteller and feel the smile her story evoked in me, as I am sure the other group members can.

Another young woman's telling of a life-threatening situation rendered the group absolutely silent in listening to this very real story. It was clear that story swapping had been instrumental in the other students' beginning to know these two women as people—at the very first class meeting.

Engaging Adolescents in Story Swapping

In spite of its value, it is not always easy to engage adolescents in story swapping, especially those with communication difficulties. Donahue (1994) described the "newcomer" profile (p. 234) that can be seen in some students with language problems or "other low-accepted children" (Putallaz & Gottman, 1981) who don't seem to understand the rules of discourse in classrooms. They might not offer stories because they are unsure of when or how to do so. A second communication style, the "immigrant" profile described by Donahue, may include the student who is not as reticent as the "newcomers," but shows inappropriate participation suggesting that this student has developed a different set of discourse rules. A third profile is presented by students who are aware of classroom participation rules, but are also aware of their own "social, linguistic and communication deficiencies" and seem to feel like "impostors" in their own classrooms (p. 244) and hesitate to join in. We hope there will be enough youngsters who feel comfortable about story swapping to provide models for others and that the stories elicited will be real enough to help adolescents join in.

The size of a group may determine the willingness of such students to participate. Adolescents who find it risky to participate in large group discussion may come forth more freely in small groups of three, in pairs of students or, perhaps, only in dialogue with an adult, away from peers. In most cases, groups of fifteen people or fewer seem to bring best participation. The challenge is to create a risk-free context by telling your own genuine stories (about you, those you know or what you have heard about) and to create a feeling of "just talking." Students will sometimes talk freely with teachers and students before-the class bell rings but not within the structure of a class, no matter how small the group. Unwittingly, as we move from "just us folks" into a teacher register in class, we instructors maintain control of the topic and create the characteristic rigid access to the conversational floor for students. We require an adherence to special conduct rules for being a speaker as opposed to a listener along with rules for procedural display (Wallach & Butler, 1994). This style change, although necessary for maintaining order in some class discussions, can hinder students' offering of their personal stories.

One experienced teacher liked this idea of story swapping but seemed unable to change "teacher talk" style and, inadvertently, made story swapping seem like a lesson rather than just talk. Students seemed to feel tested and were unable to think of something worthy to tell. One student, by his own report, never did anything interesting enough to share during this time. After story swapping was over and during a transition from one activity to another, however, this same boy commented casually that he had been chased by a cow that weekend. It was a perfect anecdote to tell, clearly a story that would have told about his experience and helped the group to know him, but he didn't see it as appropriate during story swapping. He did not realize that everyone has stories to tell.

In order to use story swapping as a viable way to know students, professionals have to develop skill in eliciting stories, particularly from reticent students. We have to create an atmosphere for sharing experiences, one that invites students to contribute. We can justify the efforts in story swapping for other reasons besides just an opportunity to listen to and know students. Story swapping can enable us to establish a shoulder-to-shoulderness (We all have stories to tell each other); to generate topics for students' writing; to develop narrative or reporting skills; and to provide one kind of listening practice, that is, listening in order to gather ideas or to find an opportunity to interrupt appropriately and tell our own story. We can use the questions in Box 5–1 to guide our observations of students in story swapping and these same questions can be used to assess students' participation in the D phase (discussion of problems) of the SPACED lessons mentioned in Chapter 2 and/or for responses in the interviews and questionnaires.

■❏ INTERVIEWS AND QUESTIONNAIRES

Interviewing can often provide an informal first step in working with adolescents. Shames and Florance (1980) discussed interviewing skills needed in their work with those who stutter. They stressed the importance of the adult's listening and actively attending during the interview, the providing of open invitations to talk along with more specific requests, and the facilitating effect of minimal encouragers such as head nods, in addition to verbally reflecting on the student's feelings and content. In addition, Shames and Florence advised the adult in the

---

BOX 5–1: *Story Swapping—Guiding Questions*

1. Does the student contribute freely? Too freely? What seems to cause the reticent student to contribute?
2. Are the stories appropriate to this setting? On the topic? An appropriate topic for the setting? Topic changed properly? With appropriate vocabulary choice for classroom? Clear to listeners or require excessive clarification? Detail? Aware of need to clarify or need questions? Right length? Aware of need to sum up?
3. Does the student persist or give up when having difficulty telling the story?
4. Does the student listen well? Sustain listening appropriately? Ask good questions?
5. What is the student's story telling style: straightforward; elaborate; with a flair?

---

interview to share his or her own experiences as a way of eliciting comments from students, although they caution us simply to "give enough to facilitate but not too much" which might shift the focus from the student to the adult (p. 32). They suggested that the adult's judicious confronting of contradictions or faulty reasoning can help students to better understand themselves and what they are saying. Finally, these authors stressed the importance of the adult's' interpreting what has been said in their restatements as a way to provide new understandings to students. These interpretations within the shoulder-to-shoulder approach also serve as a check of common understandings or premises for the collaboration.

The Learning Interview

The Learning Interview (see Box 5–2) is a good tool for obtaining an adolescent language sample, for eliciting the students' point of view, as a joint effort in beginning a collaboration, for observing pragmatic language and discourse skills, organizational problems, "meta" abilities, (See van Kleek, 1994, for discussion of metacommunication, metapragmatic and metacognition), and specific written language issues affecting the adolescent's school success.

Obtaining a Language Sample from the Learning Interview

The initial questions in the Learning Interview elicit short answers but the follow-up questions yield explanation and expansion of answers. These follow-up questions posed by an adult in the effort to clearly understand often require extended discourse from the adolescent,

BOX 5–2: *The Learning Interview*

1. What are usually your best subjects in school?
2. Why do you think these subjects are easier for you?
3. What are usually your hardest subjects?
4. What is hard about these subjects?
5. Think of a teacher who has really helped you learn? How did this teacher help you? What exactly did this teacher do that worked for you?
6. Think of a teacher whose way of teaching was not good for you. What exactly did this teacher do that did not work for you?
7. How often are you bored in class? ___ Often? ____ Sometimes? ____ Not very much? What do you do to pay better attention? Where do you sit in your classes now?
8. How often do you ask questions in class? ____ Often ____Sometimes ___Not much. What keeps you from asking a question in class? ____Embarrassed ____ Not enough time ____Teacher might say poor attention.
9. Do you catch on to new lessons easily or ____do you prefer extra explanation? Does it depend on the class?
10. When you understand something, do you usually ____ remember it or ____ do you have to go over it a lot to remember? How's your memory out of school?
11. How often are you graded down for a late or missing assignment? ____every week ____once a month ____one or two times a grading period?
12. Do you write your assignments down ____always? ____sometimes? ____never?
13. Do you usually remember to bring your books and materials ____home? ____to school?
14. Can you usually predict how well you did on a test ____(yes) or ____are you often surprised when the test grade is returned? Do you get a ____higher or ____lower grade than you predicted or ____can it be either?
15. Are you receiving any special help in ____school or ____other? When did you first start getting special help?
16. Do you have trouble understanding teacher directions? What test questions mean?
17. Can you usually explain your ideas ____easily, or is it ____hard to say what you mean? Do you have more trouble talking to ____kids or ____adults?
18. Have you ever worked with a speech language pathologist? What did you work on with the SLP?

(continued)

19. What problems do you have in reading? ____ Sounding out words?____ Finding answers to questions?____ How often do you have read something over again? ____a lot ____sometimes ____rarely. Does rereading help? ____yes ____no. Can you usually tell about what you have read? ____yes ____no. How do you feel about reading aloud in class? What have you enjoyed reading lately? Do you like ____fiction or ____nonfiction?

20. What problems do you have in writing? _____ ____Finding topics? ____Getting started in writing? ____ Writing enough? ____Spelling problems? What do you do when you need a word in your writing but you can't spell it?

21. What kind of speller are you? ____Can you memorize a list of words for a test? _____ Do you remember those words later? ____Can you find your misspellings yourself? ____Does a spell check help you?

22. Describe your math ability. ____Can you add and subtract small problems in your head or ____do you need to use your fingers? ____Have you memorized the multiplication facts? ____ Was it hard to do? ____ Do you understand: ____long division, ____fractions, ____word problems? ____ Have you had Algebra? ____How did you do in Algebra? ____Geometry?

which is not typically shown on short answer formats in formal tests. The resulting language sample can reveal a student's facility with the kinds of communication valued in classrooms. Students who can elaborate on or support their initial answers to academic questions have potential to participate more successfully than those who might know the material but are unable to show their knowledge in their comments. Students can show ability to explain, to compare their experiences in different classes, to give examples—various kinds of discourse needed in classrooms. In addition to their ability to organize their discourse, their sentence structure and speech clarity can be assessed along with fluency and voice quality. Because their answers to these questions deal with real information reflecting the students, the language and speech sample can be a realistic one.

Eliciting the Student's View

The interview may seem less threatening than most question/answer tests for students because these are not right/wrong answers. Students are informing the adult about themselves as learners and, in this effort, can show good insight. Parents are often invited to complete an intake information form in the same room during the Learning Interview and are sometimes surprised at their children's astute observations. Most adolescents do not discuss schoolwork in depth with their parents, so parents are rarely aware of what their children know about their learning. In some cases, though, a student's reports surprise their parents in a different way. For instance, one student reported in the interview, that he had a late or missing assignment "once in a while." At this remark, his mother winced visibly. I said, "It seems that your mother has a different view," and this boy looked at his mother ingenuously and said, "What?" She explained that he was regularly graded down for missing or late assignments but her son clearly did not agree with her. He seemed to be typical of those who remember having turned in many assignments here and there but without specific awareness of each day's homework for each class. Many adolescents lack natural organizational skills and seem to have a nonspecific attention style, that is, to have a general idea but not to hone in on exact detail. It is important to recognize this as a style rather than to assume that the student is lying or purposely glossing over inadequacies. There are, of course, charming, potential con artists who know very well what they have and have not done for school, but many adolescents are telling the truth as they see it and their view is vague. They need help in developing a way to specifically assess their strengths and weaknesses. The Learning Interview is one effective way to do so.

Beginning a Collaboration

The learning interview offers a quick start to the adult/student collaboration. Problems emerge and, with discussion, are clarified and possible plans begin to form. The interview process leads to individualized planning directly related to students' identified problems. The students who have good insight; who can immediately name their favorite and least favorite teachers and why, quickly distinguish themselves from those who have apparently not appreciated differences in their teachers and have no opinions on the subject. A caution is necessary here, of course. These students may be so discouraged that they have given up and written off all teachers as alike. Or, sometimes, they don't realize that they can or should have an opinion about school. Sadly, students can often quickly name their worst subject but can name no stronger subject. The interviewer must make it clear through questioning that multiple intelligences (Gardner, 1983) are being considered and that nonacademic subjects are included in this discussion. For instance, many of those who are unsuccessful in the "important" subjects have natural proclivities for art, shop, music, and sports. I make it a point, not only to include these subjects but to follow up with specific questions (What do you like best drawing, painting, sculpture ...? Do you prefer to draw with pencil, pen, markers ...? What sports do you prefer? What are your strengths and what do you have to work at?) to show that these areas have validity in a discussion of learning. Tyrel was a student (see Chapter 4) who offered his most meaningful observations in discussion of shop classes, for instance. I learned about his strengths and how angry he was that his area of expertise was not valued equally with academic subjects. His free discussion of this point suggested, perhaps, that he realized my inquiries were honest and that I valued his area of expertise, an important prerequisite for a collaboration.

Observing Pragmatic Language and Discourse Skills

The Learning Interview reveals pragmatic language skills and discourse abilities. Many adolescents come with an apparent "chip on the shoulder" and all that this implies. They open the interview with a rude question ("What's this for?") that shows that they have not chosen to come on their own and, perhaps, that they have been given little information and feel manipulated. This inappropriate style with a stranger suggests that they may also alienate teachers who, in turn, may understandably not offer the extra academic support these students need.

Sometimes a student is not angry but is inappropriately casual. For instance a high school freshman recently distinguished himself by greeting me with "Hey dude!" which startled me and seemed to horrify his mother who was sitting next to him in the waiting room. This same student who seemed to be trying to effect a "cool" style with this inappropriate greeting, however, showed an intense persistence in test taking. It was a lesson in not making snap judgments and keeping one's mind open because I assumed that his overall approach would be as flippant as his greeting.

Sometimes a student has obvious difficulty organizing sentences into clear, well ordered discourse in an attempt to answer the typical follow-up question ("What do you mean?") in the interview. After much backing-and-filling and attempts to re-compose or clarify awkward statements, the student gives up the attempt with the classic "Oh, forget it." This comment is diagnostically relevant. When I am exploring in the Learning Interview possible difficulties in expressing their ideas to others, I sometimes ask, "Do you ever know what you mean and try to say it but the other person does not seem to get it? Do you ever say, 'Oh forget it?' How often does that happen? Can you think of a time when this happened to you?" It is helpful to elicit specific instances or anecdotes that allow students to explain their answers. You can observe their narrative skill and gather examples for identifying patterns of language and behavior.

Whitmire (2000) provided a list of communication limitations of students with language-based learning disabilities (see Box 5–3). This list can be used along with the Learning Interview to guide discussion and student observations in identifying communication problems to be addressed. The list of questions in Box 5–4 can be used to discuss the communication skills identified in Box 5–3, and as assignments for directing student "research" projects for observing these skills in others. Guided observation of others and role playing can be interventions matched to specific pragmatic skills identified as lacking.

BOX 5–3: *Weak Communication Skills in Adolescents with Language-based Learning Disabilities (Adapted from Whitmire, 2000).*

1. Providing support or praise for others (Bergman, 1987).
2. Adapting one's communication to the listener's needs or feelings (Bergman, 1987).
3. Delivering tactful messages (Bliss, 1992).
4. Negotiating effectively (Gallagher, 1993).
5. Interpreting social cues (Schumaker & Hazel, 1984).
6. Understanding jokes, slang and sarcasm (Donahue & Bryan, 1984).

BOX 5–4: *Directing Discussion and/or Observation of Communication Skills*

1. Can you think of a time when you complimented a classmate or friend? Notice and write compliments you hear one classmate give another.
2. Do you find it hard to match your comments to your listener's mood? Notice and describe how a person talked in a different way or style to different people. Notice and write how a person changed the way he or she talked to the same person at different times because the listener was in a different mood.
3. Imagine that you were inviting some friends to come over to your house. Another classmate heard the plans and asked if he/she could come. What if you really did not want this person to come? How could you tell him or her that in a nice way? Notice and write down what/how someone said something unpleasant but in a nice way.
4. Do you think you are good at working with others to plan and decide things? Explain a time when you did this well. Explain a time when you did not do so well in making plans in a group.
5. Notice and write about someone who seemed to "want his/her own way" in a group planning session. Or notice when someone seems to always give in to others' choices and never gets to do what he/she wants to do.
6. Do you understand jokes or funny comments of your classmates? Notice how others respond to jokes or funny comments. Did you see someone "bluff" and act like he or she understood when you thought otherwise? Did you notice someone who looked confused when others laughed because he or she didn't "get" the joke?

Identifying Organization Problems

One can identify, in the Learning Interview, students whose primary problem seems to be organization for school. Schaeffer, Zimond, Kerr, and Farra (1990) identified six skills as most critical to school survival and four of the six seemed to directly involve organization, being on time for school, having needed materials for class, turning in work on time and following written directions. The remaining two skills included attending class every day and talking appropriately to teachers.

It is obviously important to find out, in the interview, if the student is completing homework and handing it in on time and if not, why not. It is important to distinguish true organization problems from avoidance of homework that is too difficult. When students have missing assignments and/or procrastinate in doing homework, I always ask if they have trouble making themselves complete tasks in general or if it is hard to start because they do not know how to do the schoolwork. This is certainly true for some younger students whose parents are still actively involved in homework and must reteach every subject every night. Adolescents often do not want their parents to help and/or parents are not sure if they should help older students, so homework comes to a standstill if the student does not know how to do it.

Many adolescents adopt a casual style to cover their embarrassment about school difficulties and are their own worst enemies. They don't complete work and hand it in on time. Teachers who are working hard themselves resent extending themselves for students who look as though they are not doing their part in the teaching/learning process. Students who look like they are trying (which usually means they turn in their work on time and participate in class discussions) gain sympathy and help from their teachers more readily than those who do not present themselves as hard workers.

One teenager, Kit, with severely nonfluent speech regularly responded to questions or invitations to participate in class with a nonchalant shrug and "I don't know." I suspect that some of her high school teachers misread Kit's cover-up as lack of interest or motivation. After a long collaboration period in which she maintained this same response style, I explained that we should probably stop our work on speech fluency because it was not successful. Kit returned a year later to work with me and responded to a question with her characteristic "I don't know and don't care" style accompanied by a laugh. I said, "Kit, that laugh seems close to a cry" and she did cry, which signaled her readiness to drop her defenses and enter actively into a more productive, honest collaboration. She had finally tired of spending most of her energy in covering up her severe stuttering problem and was ready to admit aloud that she had a problem, although her usual shrug and "I don't know" response was habitual and needed to be changed. Solutions were possible when Kit was ready to confront her speech problem, but one wonders how many teachers misread this casual "I don't know" style that was covering very sincere feelings.

Focusing on "Meta" Abilities

The Learning Interview allows observation of metalinguistic and metacognitive abilities (van Kleek, 1994), students' ability to consciously consider and discuss their language, thinking and learning. This awareness "allows students to acquire deliberate strategies for guiding their attention and learning processes." (Nelson, 1998, p. 7) and is an important part of an effort to help adolescents work on their own behalf.

Adolescents with academic difficulty are often practical and direct in their style and not inclined to to be "meta" on their own, but can often be directed to reflect on their thinking and learning through the interviewing process. One can tell who is already reflective and ready for problem solving as compared with adolescents who need prodding to stand back and reflect within the collaborative shoulder-to-shoulder experience.

The questions in the interview that discuss the predicting of test grades often reveal an adolescent's lack of knowledge about his or her own learning and knowing. Some students report that they can receive either a higher or lower test grade than they expected and feel that their grades are unpredictable. The questions about success in talking to others along with those about reading and writing also reveal the adolescents' language used to talk about language, their metalinguistic knowledge. Some cannot explain their difficulties because they don't know how. Questions about teachers remembered as helpful or not helpful in their learning often show students' limited metapragmatic knowledge and some students cannot provide even one specific example of ways in which a favorite teacher was helpful. Responses on the Learning Interview can reveal metalinguistic and metacognitive abilities and, for those who are not so inclined to go beyond direct experience, can provoke this kind of reflection.

Noting Possible Attention Problems

Several questions on the interview indicate possible attention problems. Students who complain about teachers talking for long periods; about being bored in class or when reading; about being unable to predict their test grades accurately; and about being graded down for missing assignments show a pattern of ineffective attention. The same students often have no preference for where they sit in a class, say that they rarely ask questions in class and do not take notes. It is easy to see that such adolescents having difficulty sustaining attention in class are also unaware that there are strategies that could help them; that they could sit within 4–6 feet of the teacher; that they could ask questions and take notes to keep themselves engaged as they listen.

The relationship between known attention problems and reading difficulties may be "confined primarily to higher level aspects of reading comprehension," (Catts & Kamhi, 1999, p. 108) and requires follow-up questioning on the interview to check expository text reading and reading of challenging literature assignments. Some students report that their

minds drift when they read or that they find it hard to sit for long periods—two indications of possible attention problems interfering with
school reading. It is always interesting to explore with adolescents the
"chicken-egg" dilemma regarding attention and reading or attention
and listening. Do they become bored, lose attention, because the reading is not making sense or does the reading not make sense because
their minds wander and they lose continuity? Are they distracted
because of noise and things they see around them, or do they lose
interest first and then notice distractions? Attention, like many other
language and learning issues, provides a productive topic for specifying problems. Those with known attention problems can discover in
these discussions that all attention problems are not equal. They need
to become experts in defining just how, when, and where their own
attention is inadequate, that is, to define the problem clearly before
solutions can be found. It is the rare adolescent with attention problems
who knows his or her problem specifically and this kind of clarification
is usually productive.

Discussing Written Language

Questions in the Learning Interview about reading, writing and
spelling are very informative. It is interesting to contrast the students'
assessments of their skills in the interview with formal test results
because many students seem unaware of their significant problems in
reading. One tenth grade student said that his reading was "average"
although his reading testing showed 3rd grade 9th month reading
level. One wonders if he was presented with extremely easy material
in his classes and that made him think his reading was adequate, or if
his "meta" skills were so limited as to cause his self-assessment to be
drastically wrong. This student was looking forward to college and,
although he had previously received special help for learning problems, had chosen to go into regular classes where he was receiving adequate to good grades, so he thought he was doing fine. His was a
severe decoding problem but his listening was a strength in classes that
offered extensive discussion. This young man needed to know his limitations, in order to prepare for more challenging classes and, particularly, for making a college plan.

Other students who have good decoding skills but poor comprehension often describe their difficulty in "remembering" what they
have read. (As Michael did, see Chapter 3) They seem unaware that
although they read the information but may not have understood the
material well enough to store it—that they had not really taken in the
information initially.

When asked the interview questions about their writing, many
students with learning problems have had little writing experience and
cannot provide many observations. Others provide responses showing
that they clearly enjoy writing, can write enough, can think of their
own topics, and so forth. Many of these students have developed

strategies to circumvent spelling problems so they have been able to continue to write. The interview reveals how much and what kind of writing experience they have had, their feelings about writing, and where in the writing process they may be having difficulty.

The discussion in the interview also helps direct the instructor to appropriate diagnostic measures. For instance, one can often guess, from the student's oral language, what to look for in their writing. Those who show a direct, unelaborated oral style may also write simply and succinctly without the complexity and more formal style expected in adolescents' writing. They may omit referents and confuse their conversational partner which would present even more of a problem in writing. If their communication style is very casual without the apparent effort to make the needed changes expected in talking to an adult they do not know well, their style in writing may also be casual and more like oral conversation than written discourse. The students' speech may show neglect of syllables or sounds in words resulting in slurred productions that are notable but do not reach the criterion for articulation disorder. They may, for instance, neglect final consonants in clusters (st, nd), produce indistinct medial tongue tip consonants (mi*dd*le, bro*th*er), omit weak syllables or sounds in challenging words ("'pecific" for "specific") and/or show word confusions (Wilmington for Wimbledon) signaling a need to explore their phonologic awareness within reading and spelling.

The Learning Interview provides a good introduction to an adolescent as student and can be a base for further exploring issues in specific classes. Lord-Larson and McKinley (1995) offered several informal questionnaires to elicit information about an adolescent's learning style, "beliefs, attitudes and misconceptions about listening " (p. 277), and attitudes about a specific class which could provide further information for identifying problems and making plans for better learning.

Single Class Interviews

One can ask students in Single Class Interviews (see Box 5–5) to describe the usual order of activities in a class; the teacher's typical method for introducing new information; the kinds of assignments the teacher favors; the teacher's grading system including penalties for late assignments and/or opportunities for extra credit; each teacher's rules or procedures for handing in assignments or for class participation along with questions about the classroom routine. Donahue (1994) also provided a helpful list of such questions from Morine-Dershimer (1985) for "assessing children's conceptions of their classroom's discourse rules" (p. 261) for elementary classrooms.

Students can be asked to observe their classes and teachers, then return with information needed to pinpoint possible problems in each class. These kinds of questions show what students already know about their classes and teachers. They also cause students to observe their

---

BOX 5–5: *Single Class Interview*

1. What is the usual routine in this class? What happens first, next, and so on?
2. Does the teacher lecture or guide discussion? If discussion, how does he/she start the discussion? What does he/she usually want you to know?
3. Is the teacher following the book closely?
4. How does the teacher want you to use the textbook? Should you read before class discussion or after? Does he/she want you to read other materials?
5. Is it hard to take notes in this class? Does the teacher use an overhead projector or the chalkboard to write notes or key words?
6. What is the usual daily homework in this class? Are there any big projects?
7. When are tests usually given? Quizzes?
8. What kind of tests does this teacher give?
9. What is this teacher's grading system?
10. Who are the best students in this class? How can you tell?
11. What do you like or dislike about this class? What is easiest and hardest in this class?
12. What would make this class easier for you?

---

classrooms and teachers more closely, which can help them learn to participate more effectively. Students with pragmatic language problems and/or poor attention particularly need this kind of discussion to help them create a context for learning content. Without this awareness, students might attend at the wrong times and/or miss pertinent information. The questions in Box 5–5 may help students think about and know their classes, teachers and textbooks

Mini-interviews focused on one class seem particularly helpful in guiding the problem solving process and personalizing it to the adolescent's current learning issues. Question 10 above, can show current assumptions about successful students which can be further explored with a mini-research assignment. Observing in class to determine when and how good students participate, exactly what they seem to know and/or ask about, for instance, may direct the less successful student to develop similar strategies for more effective preparation and participation.

The Learning and Study Strategies Inventory

The LASSI–HS Learning and Study Strategies Inventory–High School version and the LASSI for older students (Weinstein & Palmer, 1990;

Weinstein, Palmer & Schulte, 1987) is an interesting questionnaire that addresses issues in studying including attention, motivation, time management, anxiety, concentration, information processing, selecting main ideas, using study aids, self-testing, and test-taking strategies. It is a helpful tool for showing a profile of study related strengths and weaknesses, but the questions can be challenging for adolescents with language difficulties and may require clarification in order to elicit a true response. When clearly understood, however, many of the questions can provoke good discussion about how students approach schoolwork. Inherent in the questions are ideas for specific study strategies that might provide solutions for students' studying problems. For instance, questions number 23 ("I change the material I am studying into my own words"), number 26 ("I look over my notes before the next class"), and number 30 ("I stop often while reading and think over or review what has been said") would be excellent strategies to add to the routines of students who have not thought of these ideas on their own.

Parents' Observation of Language and Learning (POLL)

Parents have a unique perspective on their children's language and learning. They have watched their children and often know how they typically approach a task, what is easy and hard for them, how they communicate their ideas, and how they react to a challenge. Although we gain valuable information about adolescents from teachers' reports, test results, and their own observations in Story Swapping, the Learning Interview, Single Class Interview, and the LASSI–HS, we also need the rich observations available only to parents. Unfortunately, many professionals who work with adolescents have little time to talk with parents, beyond short interchanges in Open House, ten-minute parent-teacher conferences, short e-mail exchanges, or hurried phone conversations. The Parents' Observation of Language and Learning (POLL) (see Box 5–6) was designed as a questionnaire to elicit parents' information in an efficient form. Often parents complete the POLL to share with teachers at conference time.

BOX 5–6: *Parents Observations of Language and Learning (POLL)*

Parents: Please share your observations about your child's learning by answering the questions below. Please add any information that you feel is important.

> **1.** What is your biggest concern or question about your child's learning?

(continued)

---

2. What are your child's learning strengths? Regarding school learning? Regarding out of school learning?

3. Describe a typical homework session, that is, what the child typically has to do. List the usual subjects and tasks. What homework tasks can your child usually do without help? What tasks usually require your help? Is your child good at determining what he/she can do alone and when he/she needs your help?

4. Does your child usually understand how to do the assigned homework? Or do you have to reteach the lessons? If you have to reteach many lessons, why do you think this is necessary?

5. Does your child have homework that could or should have been completed in school? Why?

6. Does your child put off homework? ____All homework ____ Specific subjects?

7. Does your child complete homework in a reasonable time period? If not, does your child lose concentration and waste time? Explain. Does your child get "stuck" on hard work and then get off task? About how long can your child work effectively? What subjects keep his/her attention? What subjects do not?

8. Is your child inclined to check his/her work? Can he/she find errors? Can he/she correct errors? Does your child rush through work? Or does your child tend to be a perfectionist? Or give up easily?

9. Does your child avoid certain tasks? What tasks?

10. Will your child take risks in learning? Try something new? Hard? Creative?

11. What is your role in your child's homework? Explain when and how you help.

12. Have you seen your child's class notes? Do they seem complete? Legible?

13. How does your child study for tests?

14. What problems does he/she usually have on tests?

15. Does your child read and follow directions adequately?

16. What problems occur with reading assignments? How are these problems handled?

17. What problems does your child have with writing assignments? How are these problems handled? Is spelling interfering in writing? What does your child do about spelling when he/she is writing?

18. What do teachers usually say about your child? Strong points? Weak points?

(continued)

BOX 5–6: *(continued)*

19. Do you feel that your child is impulsive?

20. Can your child explain what he/she is to do for homework? Can your child explain problems with homework? Can your child explain his/her plans for projects? Does your child persist in trying to explain or give up easily?

21. Is your child organized about his/her homework? If not, explain.

22. What else have you noticed about your child's learning?

Important information can be shared through the POLL (Parents' Observations about Language and Learning) but there may be professionals who do not appreciate parents' observations about learning. One teacher complained, "If only I did not have to talk to parents, I could spend more time doing my job—teaching their children!" Another teacher was asked the question "When does a parent have the right to make a specific request for helping his or her child in the classroom?" This teacher paused and then replied, "If they are qualified ... educated" implying that parents who are not formally educated may not have valuable information about their child's learning and are, therefore, not to be heard. Add to these comments often heard as a preface to parents' remarks in school meetings, "I'm just a parent but ..." and it appears that parents' may also undervalue their perspective and their valuable observations may be lost.

When a child has special needs, of course, the parent is always included in team planning. However, there is rarely time for parents to share their ongoing observations of their children's learning. When one does have the opportunity to listen to parents, especially those whose children have extensive homework, it is remarkable what parents can tell us about their children's learning.

Teachers cannot sit beside each child as they learn so they may see only the end product without being sure of how the student figured out and executed the task. Because of social pressures in class, students sometimes do not feel free to show problems and gain help from teachers. Responses on the Learning Interview suggest that many students hesitate to ask questions in class. Fortunately or unfortunately for parents, their children complain more freely at home about learning difficulties. Parents can directly observe the process and the products of their children's learning. Parents are frustrated when teachers' comments seem to deny their concern, "All children cannot get top grades and your child's B's and C's are fine." These parents lament, "But she doesn't have any idea what my child has to go through to get those average grades!" The POLL is one practical way for parents to share their observations about learning at home. The POLL can guide, collect and present parents' observations during homework, and the

responses can add valuable information, not available elsewhere,
about adolescents' learning.

The Homework Script Questionnaire

A Homework Script Questionnaire has been useful and practical in helping students and parents identify specific homework problems that
require attention (see Box 5–7). If the student does not organize well,
both the student and the parent need to know that homework cannot be
viewed as one problem with one solution. The questionnaire illuminates
the various parts of the homework process and provides for specific discussion and planning for each step. Students who are not naturally

---

BOX 5–7: *Homework Script Questionnaire*

1. The assignment:
   Do you know when, where, how the assignments are given
   in each class?
   Are you ready with your assignment book and pencil?
   Do you write it all, accurately, legibly?
2. The materials:
   Do you get materials to class?
   Do you get materials home?
   Do you get materials back to school?
3. The homework routine:
   Is there a regular time?
   Is there a regular order of subjects?
4. Getting started:
   Do you get started on time?
   Do you understand the assignment?
   Can you teach yourself?
   Do you have materials?
5. Staying with it:
   Do you finish a task before taking a break?
   Are you distracted by hearing, seeing or thinking?
   Are you bored? Interest versus comprehension
6. Checking:
   Do you hate to check?
   Can you find/correct mistakes?
   Is there time?
7. Handing work in:
   Is there a system for keeping track of homework at home?
   Is there a system for keeping track at school?
   Writing down the assignment?

---

organized need guidance to focus on each element in homework, to identify specific problems, and to solve them one at a time.

Writing the Assignment Down

When the disorganized student does not write the assignment down this stops the homework process before it begins. Even this problem, which seems self-evident must be discussed to identify the particular difficulty. Even when a teacher gives assignments in the same way at the same time in the same place each day, there will be some students who have not noticed this routine and are never ready to write the assignment down. Some teachers assign homework immediately following the presentation of a new lesson and provide time for the students to begin the homework in class, which allows opportunities for clarifying misunderstandings. Other teachers assign the homework at the end of the class with no time for questions. There are also teachers who become caught up in discussion, forget to give the homework until after the bell has rung, and frantically call out the assignment as students are leaving because the teacher knows that an upcoming test has already been typed and includes information from the assignment. Whatever the style of the teacher, students need to plan to have their assignment book ready at the appropriate time.

Many adolescents do not realize that teachers cannot always solve their learning problems, can even cause problems because of their own style, and that students must find their own solutions. Those who assume that academic skill is an inborn talent, seem surprised that they contribute to their own school success by problem solving at these times. Knowing when the assignment is usually given helps one prepare for writing it down, but one also needs to have pencil and assignment book ready to do so and this may require a conscious plan. Parents often assume that simply telling their child to "Be ready" will suffice and need to appreciate that, for the disorganized adolescent, conscious planning may be necessary even for such a small thing as having a pencil with them in class.

The Homework Script Questionnaire identifies specific homework problems and provides an opportunity to develop a plan, monitor the plan and revise it quickly if it is not working. Students learn that their plan must be memorable, that is, they cannot just depend on good intentions alone. They must make a plan that they will definitely remember to follow. One student's plan included sewing Velcro on the inside of the handle of his book bag, which he would feel when he carried his bag, and a fluorescent patch on the top of the bag, two signals that he understood reminded him to put his assignment book and pencil out on the desk at the beginning of every class. This plan seemed like a good one but it did not work. He still forgot to get his pencil and assignment book out so another plan was devised. He chose a good friend in each class and visualized this friend saying something embarrassing about him before class. The only way he could prevent such an episode in this plan was to put his assignment book out as he entered

each class. In order to make this imaginary scenario memorable, this
student was encouraged to elaborate on and exaggerate the threatened
remark and the feelings he would have in that eventuality. This
discussion emphasized the need for planning consciously in order to
be ready to write when the teacher gave the assignment, to monitor the
plan and to revise it in a way what would ensure it would work.

Writing the Assignment Accurately

Those students who consistently write their assignments at the right
time still face the possibility that their account may not be accurate or
complete and they may not discover this problem until they try to do
the homework or until papers are graded down because of a missing
element. Specific plans need to be devised, monitored and made habitual to avoid this problem. Many students use strategies such as calling
a friend to clarify an assignment, which is sometimes necessary, but
they never seem to plan ahead to avoid this problem in the first place.
Students and teachers can collaborate by having someone restate the
assignment in class so everyone can check their understanding and
accuracy. Weekly checks of grades can guide attention to when and
what was missed in writing down the assignment. The student can be
engaged in writing assignments to dictation then comparing with the
original to determine what was missed and to direct attention to the
important parts of assignments.

Utilizing Tracking Systems

Tracking systems in which teachers or counselors view and check
assignment books daily are often used to ensure that students write
assignments completely and accurately. Unfortunately, even though
many students continue to need this kind of assistance throughout
school, too often it is discontinued after elementary school. Many adolescents who are not naturally talented in devising organizational systems on their own need this kind of guidance and support through
high school and college.

For a homework tracking plan to work, someone needs to monitor
it at school and at home, to notice quickly when the student is not following the plan, and collaborate with the student in identifying the
problem. If the student is embarrassed by having to check with the
teacher publicly, then the plan is not a good one and needs to be
altered. The same is true if the plan depends on a very disorganized
student to remember on his/her own to come and be checked. If students had that ability they probably wouldn't need a conscious plan! It
is rare that this flaw in the plan is detected because it is usually
assumed that the student is just "not taking responsibility." One middle school student clearly had difficulty with organization and was losing ground in school, not because of difficulty in conceptualizing new
information, but because he was not handing in the work. In this case,

he regularly completed homework but lost track of it between home and school. His mother was asked if the school had made attempts to monitor his assignment book and she replied, "Oh, yes but I never saw the book after the first week." Neither the school nor the parent realized the need to follow up on the initial plan to see if it was working. The plan, for this child, was ultimately revised with the school counselor and student developing a way for him to remember to come to her office to check the homework each day.

For students with known attention problems or learning differences such a tracking plan needs to be written into their learning plan with weekly reports between school and home to ensure successful implementation. High school and college students with organization problems need creative planning to ensure that they monitor with less assistance. Specific periodic times for evaluating the plan should be required to allow for adjustments to be made before serious problems develop. Students need this support as many have had limited experience in making and/or following plans over sustained periods. They are learning a new skill and need a collaborator to work with them in developing effective organizational habits.

Managing School Materials

Remembering to take home the appropriate books and other materials requires the same kind of problem solving and many parents remind (nag?) students daily or even return to school for needed materials in their children's elementary years. Some procure an extra set of textbooks for home and, in extreme cases, this may be necessary; however, parents and students should be guided in devising plans for managing materials for study. Some schools limit locker visits presumably to direct students to obtain materials for several classes at once rather than to race to their lockers between every class. One student complained that if he were late for his second period class again, he would be punished. Even though his first two classes were side by side and his locker was on the other side of the school, this student did not realize that there was an alternative to his racing to and from his locker between these two classes. For this student and others, it has been helpful to plan an early morning locker visit to retrieve materials for all morning classes, perhaps morning books and folders colored coded for quick identification ("Get all the materials with red dots on your early locker visit"). The student, in this plan, returns to the locker midday and exchanges morning for afternoon materials ("Blue dots") and makes a final visit after school *with assignment book in hand* to guide selection of books to take home. As with any new plan, this one has to be clear to the student ("Let's review the plan. Explain it to me so I can be clear about what you intend to do"), and it has to seem plausible given the student's personality and particular needs ("Does this seem like it will work? Is there any part that doesn't feel right—that doesn't fit you? Are there any changes that need to be made—even small

---

BOX 5–8: *General Principles for Problem Solving in Homework*

- Identify a specific problem.
- Make a memorable plan that fits the student.
- Try out the plan and check for flaws.
- Revise the plan.
- Practice consciously until the plan is habitual.

---

changes?"). Once devised and understood, the plan has to have a trial period to identify problems and/or changes that need to be made. For instance, the student may need some of the morning books for an afternoon study period so the mid-day exchange may need to be adjusted. The plan then has to become habitual and automatic.

Parents and students need to understand that just having a plan does not ensure that it will be workable or that it can be easily learned. The principles for problem solving with homework are similar throughout the process: identify the specific problem, make a plan that is memorable and fits the student, try it out and check for flaws, revise, and practice it consciously to make it a habit (see Box 5–8).

Avoiding Homework

Many students do not have a regular time set aside for homework and seem to study on an as-needed basis, which becomes a problem as the work load increases in middle school, high school and college. Almost every student, no matter how academically inclined, will encounter a challenging subject or teacher at some stage in school and need a more regular study program in order to keep up with the daily work. When there is extensive information to learn, they will need daily review to make studying for tests easier. One student seemed to feel he could not be tied down to a schedule; that he simply did not operate this way and preferred to keep his options open. This was difficult and almost stopped the collaboration, but it was a good opportunity to apply the shoulder-to-shoulder approach. The student was asked to suggest an alternative plan that included flexibility for his style but with the understanding that a weekly report from the school would show whether his plan was working, that is, whether he was keeping up to date with homework. Rather than trying to impose a more effective plan when adolescents are resistant allows them to try out their own ideas which sometimes do work. For instance, there are students who use music or TV as a masking noise to block out other distractions during study, and parents worry because they feel one can only study in a quiet atmosphere. Those students could try studying under their favored noisy conditions with a weekly check of homework and grades and the understanding that, if their system does not serve them well, they will then try the quiet approach favored by their parents.

The students whose major problem is procrastination need to find out why they are postponing homework. Perhaps they don't understand the work. In that case, they may need a plan that requires previewing information before class to facilitate listening comprehension, or to tape record class discussions and lectures to allow for a second chance at understanding, or working with a tutor or a study buddy.

Many students begin their work on time but give up quickly when an assignment seems too hard ("She didn't teach us this. I hate it when she says 'Figure it out on your own.' That's her job! There's no way I can learn this if she doesn't teach it."). Discussion may reveal the view that if one is not born talented at learning, little can be done and so these students have not explored strategies such as looking back at previous problems to help with new problems in math, looking for key words in the index in order to locate information quickly in text, reading aloud to direct attention to ideas, and so on.

Identifying and discussing avoidance of homework, can reveal learning problems and insufficient skills along with misconceptions about study. Too often the problem solving process stops when the adolescent's frustration is viewed as "just not trying." Parents need to realize that this frustration may signal a need for help in identifying and solving problems surrounding schoolwork. That student may need to work within a collaborative problem solving partnership.

Too Much Time Required for Homework

Some students maintain a regular study time and spend hours on homework every day, but continue to do badly in school. It is important to explore this problem before the student gives up. It is easy to see how angry a student must feel after doing more work than others who receive higher grades.

One student was attending an accelerated program in which he could graduate from high school at age 15. Transferring to this school was his idea and his parents were encouraged that he seemed motivated for the first time to do well in school. He was reportedly spending five hours on homework every night, which confirmed his good intentions but he was having little success so his parents began questioning the appropriateness of this particular school for their son. Because he wanted to stay in the program, problem solving was definitely needed to increase his study effectiveness. Discussions of this student's studying revealed that he had no difficulty beginning his work but was easily distracted and had difficulty maintaining his best effort. Therefore, very little of the actual homework time was productive. We reviewed this student's usual order of study to see if changes were indicated. He attended to his hardest subjects first, and this seemed to be a good decision—to do the difficult work while he was fresh. In this young boy's case, however, it seemed more effective for him to complete the work for only one difficult class and then to reward himself with an easy or

favorite subject rather than expending all his energy on the hard subjects.
We decided to include planned break times also.

Advice to Students or Know Yourself and Plan. Know your body. Find
out how long you can sit and plan accordingly. Allow for both mini-
breaks and major breaks but be sure to finish a task before you break. You
have to become your own parent and nag yourself to finish the work
before the fun. Then plan the breaks intelligently. Know yourself. If you
have trouble coming back after a long break, think of a way to be sure
you will not waste time. Set a timer and think of a reward to give
yourself for being in your chair ready to study before the bell rings. Be
your own boss and make plans for yourself. Plan mini-breaks but make
it a rule that you will be tethered to the chair during these breaks. You
can move, and you probably need to, but imagine that you can only
move an arm's length from the chair. Does this plan make sense to you?
If so, write these plans down so your parents will know that you are trying something different to make your studying better.

Reading Assignments

Some students avoid reading assignments and depend almost exclusively on class discussion for their learning. If they have serious decoding problems, a responsive plan might include recorded texts with
guided help in learning to use them, having a notetaker in class, and
tape recording class discussions with help in using notes and listening
to the tape at night (See Michael's example, Chapter 3).

If the problem is reading comprehension this often goes unidenti-
fied or is not directly addressed. Adolescents who can read the words
but not the meanings don't know what to do, which makes reading
unsatisfying so then they avoid it.

At about fourth grade, new vocabulary is acquired primarily
through reading (Miller & Gildea, 1987), so those who avoid reading
lag behind habitual readers in their vocabulary development and, presumably, the world knowledge associated with new words. A negative
spiral can begin because for those with reading difficulty reading
makes no sense at times due to unfamiliar vocabulary, so the student
doesn't read. Because they don't read, they acquire fewer new vocabulary words and related knowledge to aid comprehension, which contributes to further difficulty in reading attempts.

Teachers regularly address vocabulary, but too often the emphasis
is on finding and copying definitions that are then matched to new
words and memorized. Presenting vocabulary in this way implies that
a definition accompanied by one example sentence will make the word
meaningful and allow students to use that word effectively. Unfortunately, it is not always clear how to use a word without hearing and/or
reading it repeatedly, supported by context.

I am reminded of a middle-aged woman who was extremely motivated to improve her vocabulary. When a miscue was noted in her

reading, she acknowledged this by saying, "I'm cognizant, I'm cognizant." She seemed to know something about the meaning of this word but to be unaware of the way to use it correctly.

Defining words is one way to learn them but an incomplete understanding often results. We need to address vocabulary as one way to increase comprehension in reading or listening and to facilitate effective expression. Adolescents will be better served, however, when new words are encountered in a rich supportive language context followed by hearing/seeing those words used in a variety of sentences expressing a similar meaning. Many adolescents have not broadened their understanding of "new and subtle meanings" for familiar words (Nippold, 1988, p. 44) and they need help in appreciating new meanings for known words. In any case, introduction to new words or new meanings for known words in a variety of contexts can make the dictionary definitions more usable. Of course, students with limited skill in language learning and/or in memory will also need many opportunities to hear and use new words to truly incorporate them into their working vocabulary.

One parent brought in a note from her child's teacher asking her to "help your child with comprehension." This student didn't know what to do in order to comprehend more effectively on his own, the parent did not know what to do to help at home, and, it appeared from the general nature of the note, that the teacher did not know exactly what to suggest. Specific strategies for comprehension need to be explored with students. Simply telling adolescents or their parents to "work on comprehension" will not help if no one knows what to do.

The adolescent with comprehension problems needs help in learning how to "warm up" for reading (see Chapter 7) both expository text and fiction. Invariably, adolescents who are struggling in school approach assigned readings by simply opening the book and starting to read without noting the topic, without realizing the need to evoke old information by looking over the chapter first to guide their comprehension of new information. They don't think to become grounded in a short story or novel by consciously noting early in their reading the basic plot, the setting, the time period, the characters and the role of each character in the assumed plot. These same students may be very good at social reconnaissance, that is, looking over the crowd to see what kind of party it is and who is there so they can have a sense of "what's happening" before they begin participating, but they need to be directed in applying a similar prediction strategy in school reading. Because they don't warm up to the overall topic first, adolescents without natural comprehension skills are often reduced to memorizing isolated facts without appreciating how these facts relate to each other or to the overall topic (see Brent in the Prologue). Plans for these students need to address immediate homework needs along with acquisition of long-term comprehension strategies such as "warming up."

Specific Homework Solutions

Specific homework solutions might require an adult collaborator to model reading of expository text chapters by 1) creating a web of topics and subtitles, and 2) reading the summary and adding information to the web. This visual representation of the title and the subtitles with major points from a summary can be described as a working mental file, "a warm-up" for reading. The adult can then guide the reading of each section of the chapter, taking turns with the student, stopping after each paragraph to identify the topic and the main point being made about the topic ("Okay. What is this paragraph about? What point are they making about the topic? In other words, why did they write this paragraph? Okay, I'll write that point down in key words, a statement or a question form to use for studying."). This plan for reading a chapter should be modeled, practiced with supervision and gradually incorporated into the student's conscious, independent reading script with periodic checks of understanding . ("Now, I want to be sure that you are clear on what we have been doing. How would you explain what we do when you have a new chapter to read in social studies? Tell what we do at each step and why. What do you do to warm up first? Why? What do you need to ask yourself about paragraphs? Why? ").

Checking and Returning Homework

Many students do their homework regularly but their grades suffer because they hate to check their work. They may be those who need novelty and are quickly bored with old information. Or they might include students like Paul (described in Chapter 4) who are frustrated because they cannot find their mistakes. In any case, not checking their work causes students to lose points and they need a plan that overcomes their resistance to checking their work. ("Here's another of those cases where you have to become your own parent, teacher or boss and create a plan that ensures that you will check—not just the intention to check, but a specific plan to make sure that you will check.").

Some checking plans (see Box 5–9) stress finishing all the homework, taking a break and then a having a checking step that must be completed before a favorite TV show or other desirable or habitual activity. Other plans add a checking step after each subject is completed because checking everything at once seems too time consuming. Students like Paul may need to ask a parent to check the work first and write the total number of errors noted. The student then checks the paper keeping a daily record of the percentage of errors found (How many of the total errors did the student find each day?). As students identify their errors, they will become vigilant for specific error types.

The student who completes and checks the homework but fails to hand it in may need to find a spot at home for all school materials, a "home locker," and to invite someone at home to reinforce the use of this

---

BOX 5–9: *Suggested Plans for Checking Homework*

1. Finish all homework—take a break—check work before a favorite TV show.
2. Check each subject's work as completed.
3. Ask parent or sibling to check first. Keep record of the percentage of errors you find.
4. Put homework in a folder and put the folder in a special place (your home locker).

---

locker until habits are established for always putting finished homework materials there and for collecting materials from the locker before leaving for school. An innovative plan for one student required that he announce in a loud voice when he had finished each subject's homework and had placed it in his homework folder. After the last task, he then found a "witness" to verify that he had put his bookbag in his home locker.

Whatever the student's pattern of strengths versus weaknesses, it is important to appreciate that homework is not one problem that can be "fixed" in one step. There are many steps to consider in solving homework problems, and it is important to make a continuing effort to specify problems and make personalized, workable plans. Students who develop successful plans for completing and handing in homework will be more likely to receive assistance or at least the benefit of the doubt from teachers who can see that the students are doing their part in the learning process. ("Remember, if you show the teacher that you are doing your part by turning in homework, the teacher will be more likely to favor you when your work is hovering between two possible grades!").

Teacher Observation Questionnaire

Information from teachers is, of course, very important for understanding an adolescent's language and learning. It can be elicited in a variety of oral or written forms but a Teacher Observation Questionnaire (see Box 5–10) can allow teachers to reflect about a particular student before conferences.

Teachers' observations tell us something different about an adolescent than do the reports of parents and student. To collaborate well, professionals need to appreciate the richness of these various perspectives and to mine all these sources.

Multiple Intelligence Profiling

Creating a profile of multiple intelligences with the student has been suggested as a good way to identify problems and guide the making of

---

BOX 5–10: *Teacher Observation Questionnaire*

Re: John Dough

Date_____

Permission signature_____

Parent signature_____

John and his parents have given permission for me to learn about his performance and participation in your class to inform our working together to improve his language and learning skills. Please complete the following checklist and add any observations we have omitted.

1. How would you describe John as a student in your class?
2. What do you think John needs to do to improve his work in your class?
3. What is John's attention like in your class? Is he able to sustain his listening? Can he maintain his focus during individual or small group work? Does he attend well in whole group discussion?
4. Does John seem to know the usual routine in your class? Is he ready when you begin your lessons? Is he ready when you give oral directions or assignments?
5. Does John seem organized in your class? Does he have needed materials? Does he hand in homework on time?
6. How does John participate in oral discussion? Does he make appropriate comments? Does he add to the information? How often does he comment? Are his comments appreciated by others? Does he ask questions? How often? Are they appropriate questions? Does he answer questions in a timely manner? In a clear fashion? Do you see notable differences in John's participation in whole group, small group or paired learning situations?
7. What can you tell about John's reading? Is he willing to read aloud? How well does he read orally? Does he seem to comprehend?
8. What can you tell about John's writing? Can he generate ideas for topics? Can he narrow topics to make them workable? Is he willing to write? Can he write enough? Does he express his ideas clearly? Does spelling cause him difficulty in writing? Is he avoiding challenging words because of spelling?

---

plans (Miller, 1990; 1993). School subjects can be listed along with nonacademic activities and the student can be guided in creating bar graphs to show relative strengths and weaknesses in various classes and activities ("On a scale of 1–10, how would you rate yourself in math ... in English ... in sports ... in art?"). Parents, teachers, SLPs or other adult collaborators can also create bar graphs showing their view of the student's profile. Scores from standardized tests can be shown in this same way and these various perspectives can be compared by making transparencies of the graphs and superimposing them one on the other. This might be a good way to discover how the student is being perceived and is perceiving him/herself. This kind of graphic representation can clearly point out areas of weakness where planning needs to be done. The strengths will be obvious and ways can be explored for using strengths to shore up weaknesses. Miller reported (personal communication) for instance, that a child who was failing his computer class revealed in his profile a strength in organizing his extensive baseball card collection on his home computer, a system he tended weekly. In joint planning, his computer teacher, who was also a baseball card buff suggested using the student's baseball card system in computer class and this child began to improve. Graphic representations like these or displaying scores on a normal curve graph allow students to better understand their strengths and weakness and create a good focus for planning.

Analyzing Student School Work

To learn about adolescents' language and learning it is essential that one review the work they are doing in school. Looking at their tests, for instance, can show patterns such as skipping questions, getting mixed up when using answer sheets, apparently losing concentration and losing points at the end of a test. Examining question–answer matches can reveal misreading or partial reading of questions. Discussion can show instances in which the student actually knew the answer but misread the question.

Sometimes students can increase their grades dramatically when given the same test orally, suggesting effects in written tests of decoding problems, language comprehension problems, poor planning under time constraints, problems in spelling or handwriting, and so forth. Discussion of when and how adolescents study for tests can show a variety of problem areas. Students who do well on daily work but not on tests need to collaborate to check their accurate reading of test questions, the accuracy and clarity of their class notes, their ability to ferret out important information from class discussion and their reading, their attention to teachers' directions about what to study for the test, and the possible effects of anxiety during tests. Many students never look at their class notes until the night before a test and are overloaded with information. Reviewing their notes can also show incomplete sentences or disordered information, illegible notes, and/or language that the student wrote accurately and clearly but does not understand.

Reviewing Study Guides

Completed study guides in which students find and write information can show ability to comprehend questions and to locate pertinent information. Asking students to demonstrate how they find the information for the study guide often reveals their leafing through the chapter rather than finding a question's key word in the index to quickly locate the appropriate page. Sometimes they seem to match a key word from a question to that same key word in a sentence from the chapter, and then write that sentence without apparently checking its sense or relevance. Listening to students explain the information after they have completed the study guide can show their memorizing of isolated facts without placing the information in the context of the overall topic or related facts. Asking students how they would study the information can show their strategies. Many students reply that they "go over it" without indications that they check their understanding or their retention of information. One student, in such a discussion, explained that she did not have to know what the chapter was about or what the guiding question meant. She clearly felt that she should simply memorize the answers that had been discussed in class and written down for her. This was important information to guide this student in more effective processing of information in homework.

Checking Textbook–Student Fit

Using the students' textbooks to observe their reading can show when the text is too difficult because of vocabulary and assumed background knowledge, word decoding requirements, sentence level and discourse level language demands, and so forth. It is helpful to construct an informal cloze test using a 300-word passage from the second page of a new chapter in the student's text. We copy the passage, use a marker to cover every ninth word, number each created blank, copy the marked, numbered passage, ask the students to read the first page of the chapter, then to read the marked passage and write on a separate sheet a probable word for each blank. We judge the students' word choices on the basis of fit with the overall topic and grammatical fit within the sentence. Students whose accuracy in word predictions is below instructional level (75–89% correct) on this measure will need accommodations such as recorded textbooks or inclusion in a language experience group in which the book is read aloud to them, discussed, then summarized by the group and rewritten in their own words.

Discussion with the student can reveal misunderstandings about how to use their textbook. For instance, many students do not realize that reading the chapter is necessary. They assume that their responsibility is only to find answers to questions at the end of chapters or in a study guide. One student reported that he did not have to read the textbook. He said that the teacher was covering material from the textbook but he did not have to read the book. Even though this student was not doing well in the class, he had not realized that reading the material might support his understanding of class discussion. One has to check the textbook and discuss the use of the book with teachers, because they may be dissuading students from reading a book that is difficult or poorly written. Some teachers have become discouraged when students are unable or unwilling to read the books independently and stop assigning the reading. They may depend on students' reading aloud in class, which may not help a student who cannot follow along when the reading is difficult. A teacher may also assume that students know, without being told, to read the book in addition to listening in class and studying their notes. In any case, adolescents' use of their textbooks needs to be investigated in order to help them become more proficient students.

Checking Language Issues in Writing

Writing samples, particularly rough drafts, can show language strengths and weaknesses and add relevance to the results of standardized tests. A limited sample of writing one day within a time constraint in a measure such as the *Test of Written Language-3* (Hammill & Larsen, 1996) or on the two sentence level measures on the *Test of Adolescent and Adult Language, 3* (Hamill, Brown, Larsen & Wiederholt, 1996) may not show the students' typical writing, their best writing when they have time for reflection, or the kind of writing their teachers are assigning. Discussing writing assignments with students is very important to show their understanding of what teachers expect, first. There was one conscientious high school junior who lost many points on an important term paper because he misunderstood the teacher's directions. He did not clarify his understanding because he was sure he knew what to do. It was unclear then, if this student's grade reflected his writing ability or his comprehension of directions. It is not always possible, but would be helpful to see samples of writing for the better students and to discuss the rubric for grading papers with the teacher in order to evaluate a student's work in the context of classroom expectations. For many adolescents it is necessary to check their understanding of the rubric, to teach the rubric explicitly using student writing samples to show each requirement, and to guide their use of the rubric to check their own writing.

Discussion of his or her writing process can reveal a student's schema for writing. One very concrete and succinct language user regularly lost points on essay answers. His teacher asked him during one test to "tell me more, Jack" and he did. He apparently knew more but did not realize exactly what was required in an essay answer. Other students would not be so easily "fixed" and might need modeling and guided practice using a written set of guidelines to produce more expanded and complete written answers.

Some students write too little and cannot expand. Some students ramble and write too much without ever getting to the point. Balancing information with the reader in mind requires pragmatic language ability that may be revealed in writing. The writer may have difficulty taking the reader's perspective and responding accordingly. They may have the teacher in mind and assume she or he knows the information so it does not have to be told. The student can have the reader's perspective in mind but be unable to organize the information as evidenced by much backing and filling or redundancy.

Many adolescents' writing looks immature. They write little, use simple sentences and low-level vocabulary. It is important to try to elicit information orally about a topic within the student's interest and knowledge base to get the best language sample. Asking them to write that piece down may produce their best language. Some students do not have to be extremely engaged and can produce passable language even when writing about the teacher's assigned topic rather than their own, but others may "go through the motions" and not show their best language unless it is personally relevant. They have to be able to do both—write on their own interesting topics and reveal their real voice in writing, and comply with less interesting topics assigned by teachers. To assess their actual writing ability, we have to see samples of both kinds of writing.

■ SUMMARY

This chapter has presented a variety of informal ways to gain information about adolescents' language and learning. The tools described allow adolescents to inform us about their learning, offering insights that can lead to personalized planning. Story swapping elicits very real language reflecting adolescents' experiences, narrative style and ability and showing skills necessary for communicating to a naive listener or for functioning within a group discussion. Follow-up questions in the Learning Interview such as asking youngsters to "talk more about how that particular teacher helped you" can elicit specific examples that identify patterns in communication and learning. These extended discussions that are focused on the adolescent's information also encourage and show the ability to elaborate beyond basic sentences, a necessary skill for successfully showing one's knowledge or perspective in higher level classes. Single Class Interviews allow adult collaborators to understand the youngsters' view of their specific learning needs relative to class requirements. These interviews provoke metacognitive and metalinguistic awareness. The LASSI–HS can show strengths and weakness in studying and the questions suggest specific strategies for improvement. The POLL and Homework Script Interviews provide the rich observations of parents over a lifetime of supervising home studying and can guide specific planning for improved language processing for school. The Teacher Observation Questionnaire tells us about the adolescent's ways of proceeding within a classroom. Multiple intelligence profiling allows a visual representation of strengths and weaknesses showing the perspectives of the student, the parent and the teacher which can be discussed along with standardized test results. Reviewing and discussing artifacts from students' class-work is critical for identifying relevant problems to be addressed. Their own tests, reading of texts and school writing assignments can show relevant problems that need to be addressed and strengths that may not show in standardized measures. These tools provide information but also support the communication within a collaboration leading to informed planning for the benefit of adolescents in need of help.

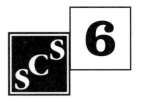

Formal Testing of Adolescents' Language and Learning

This chapter presents issues surrounding formal testing of adolescents' language and learning. There is discussion of formal tests for professionals to use or peruse in the effort to better understand the language and learning of adolescents and to help adolescents better understand themselves The list of instruments is not exhaustive, but includes tests for intelligence, executive function, perceptual and motor abilities, memory, attention, and oral and written language.

Individual testing provides opportunities to observe the way an adolescent or young adult proceeds in taking a test but valuable diagnostic information is lost if an examiner records only correct or incorrect responses. This chapter describes ways to gain diagnostic information beyond that implied by standard scores alone.

■□ APPRECIATING THE ADVANTAGES AND DISADVANTAGES OF FORMAL TESTING

Testing has become front-page news. With the introduction of high-stake, widespread testing, there is lively discussion among professionals and the general public about formal versus informal testing. Muma (1978) cautioned us long ago about the limitations of standardized language testing, favoring a more functional assessment in its place. Others have also observed that results of formal testing alone rarely result in appropriate intervention goals (Prigatano et al., 1986; Szekeres, Ylvisaker, & Cohen, 1987). Formal tests do not assess awareness of cognitive deficits, and rarely elicit spontaneous strategies and their effects on functional task performance or the effect of strategic suggestion on performance. Efficiency in the learning of significant amounts of information over extended periods of time cannot be measured in a standardized test format nor can the ability to generalize newly acquired skills to novel situations. Effects of real life stress (time pressure, performance expectations and interpersonal stress) on concentration and problem solving or ability to shift attention as needed is rarely observed within discreet formal testing, although these observations are critical for helping adolescents function on the job and in school (Szekeres, Ylvisaker, & Cohen, 1987). There is also the consideration that people can sometimes perform better in structured testing than in real life situations (Baxter, Cohen & Ylvisaker, 1985; Jennett & Teasdale, 1981; Prigatano et al., 1986) and the opposite can also be true—that some are not good test takers but perform better on their jobs, in school or in social situations than their test scores would predict.

Patricia B. Launer (1994) in responding to a question posed by Butler and Wallach (1994) warned against the two most "profound pitfalls" in using standardized measurements: irresponsible consumerism and inaccurate interpretation. She suggests we evaluate tests for their statistical validity and reliability, of course, but also for their relevance to the student in question (McCauley & Swisher, 1984). Launer provides reasons why we should not rely exclusively on standardized tests: 1) tests do not reflect real communication including appropriate language use; 2) they focus on specific skills in specific ways that may not transfer to real situations; 3) they cause anxiety and may underestimate ability; 4) they are not appropriately interactive and view the student as the responder only; 5) they allow for little creatively or flexibility in scoring; 6; they do not reflect communication in classroom; and 7) standardized tests are often not sensitive to cultural differences.

Curriculum based language assessments have been devised to address concerns about standardized test scores not reflecting actual classroom requirements and/or optimum performance (Nelson, 1989, 1998; Marston, 1989; Shinn, 1989; Tucker, 1985). Outcome based learning goals have also been developed in an attempt to make observations more appropriate but have drawn fire from those who question the validity of what can seem like subjective assessments. There continues to be a need for the public to see measures showing statistical comparison to others of the same age or grade. The need to be accountable for spending extra funds and/or for justifying program approaches clearly requires "numbers" and comparisons. Parents and adolescents themselves are accustomed to scores and grades and seem uncomfortable or confused when performance is described only in qualitative terms. Standardized measures can contribute to collaborative discussions and problem solving and, in spite of their limitations, can help answer initial questions ("Is the adolescent in trouble? How far below expectations does he fall?") and ongoing questions about progress ("How's she doing? Is she catching up?").

Rourke (1994), has argued extensively for standardized tests and "measures presented in a standardized fashion" for neuropsychologic assessment (Rourke & Adams, 1984; Rourke et. al., 1983; Rourke, Fisk & Strang, 1986) in order to compare results with developmental norms and in repeated assessments. Rourke (1994) noted the difficulty of replicating qualitative measures or being able to verify through informal measurement the efficacy of treatment/intervention methods.

■□ USING BOTH FORMAL AND INFORMAL TESTING FOR ADOLESCENTS' BENEFIT

It seems clear that we gain information through both formal and informal diagnostic means. Standardized tests give us base lines and one kind of measure of change over time along with comparisons to peers, but classroom-based assessments, observations within a variety of other situations by a variety of observers along with self-reports are necessary to verify the standardized results with the adolescent's reality. It is also important to put all testing in perspective. We need testing to help define problems in starting shoulder-to-shoulder collaborations and to focus on progress along the way, but in reality, all teaching and learning is diagnostic. We don't just observe processes and products during testing time. Throughout the process of working with adolescents we identify problems and make plans, observe and note strengths, weakness, strategies, patterns. Formal testing is one part of the process.

Observing Adolescents During Test Taking

Within formal testing there are meaningful observations that can be made beyond that implied by standardized scores. One can identify in testing, attentiveness versus distractibility, organized versus fragmented thinking and expression, flexibility versus perseveration, deliberate versus impulsive manner, and abstract versus concrete thinking. (Szekeres et al., 1987, p. 126). It is also helpful to note during testing if and how comprehension is affected by an increase in length and complexity of the material (Cohen, 1986).

An observational tool to accompany formal testing (see Box 6–1) was developed by the author and reviewed for suggestions by professionals who regularly evaluate adolescents: a psychologist (Thomas McCann, Ed.D.) a vocational evaluator (Ed Ryan) and a social worker turned school counselor, (Hope Conroy, M.S.W., L.C.S.W.). The assumption underlying this effort was that one often gains important information about an adolescent's learning style by observing how the student takes tests. Standard scores are given more meaning when one knows how they were achieved, in other words how the student approached the tasks. For instance, students who are hesitant to risk will show you only what they are absolutely sure about and will not reveal concepts that are forming. Nor will they show good logic in spite of wrong answers. The fact that these kinds of students are so hesitant to guess suggests that their scores may be minimal estimates of what they actually know. The score can reflect what they usually "do" but not what they "can do." Impulsive students, on the other hand, may produce wrong responses because of their quick responding. These students' scores may also show what they typically "do" because of their style, but not what they "can do" if they were more reflective. Observing students in action during testing provides good information about their learning style and makes the resulting score more meaningful.

Responses to Directions and Questions

During formal testing, we can observe the adolescent's ability to follow oral and written directions. There are those who seem to "catch on" to the task easily and seem confident from the beginning. There are those who seem unclear about the directions and to figure out the task only after several test items have been administered. This is an important observation as standardized testing procedures constrain the examiner's presentation of directions. An adolescent who finds test directions difficult and requires extra examples provided by the first several test items will probably have difficulty with directions in class in addition to losing points on standardized tests as he or she learns the task. In some cases, the adolescent who needs to be particularly sure or needs many examples to understand the language of directions may have the knowledge inherent in the test but the examiner may discontinue the test before a basal understanding has been established. In these cases, the score reflects receptive language difficulties, regardless of the intent of the test.

Question–answer matches throughout interviews are very important in determining receptive abilities. One must notice and then differentiate those who do not understand even with repetition from those who seem inattentive or nervous on the first presentation but clearly understand on the second. There are also adolescents who make "premature cognitive commitment" (Langer, 1989, p. 22) to their first assumptions based on inadequate information and answer inappropriately because they did not hear the entirety of the question. This group stays with their first answer in spite of new information. There are also those who make impulsive first guesses and then self-correct but persist in having to correct because of their quick responses. We must assess willingness to risk as it affects students' responding to directions and questions in formal testing. For those who are hesitant to risk, we only see those answers about which they are very sure and never get to see their problem solving. To make formal test results usable, we need to notice mismatches in question–answer or direction–response and to try to understand why they occur,

---

BOX 6–1: *Learning Style Observations During Testing*

1. Does the student seem motivated to show his/her best abilities? If challenged will he/she persist at a task? Will he/she push him/herself if necessary? Does this student seem to have high goals? Too high?

2. Do responses seem impulsive? Does the student begin before oral directions are completed? Does the student "speed up" in his/her work?

3. Does the student seem to attend to the "big picture" but not to the parts of the task? Or does the student seem to consider the parts without noting the overall idea?

4. Does the student predict with a reasonable logic but neglect to confirm the predictions by checking (may vary with different kinds of tasks)?

5. Does the student seem overwhelmed with the amount of information and/or to give up when tasks become difficult? Is the student a risk taker?

6. Is the student a good problem solver? Verbally and nonverbally? Does he/she seem to have a plan or to respond randomly? Does he/she seem to have optional strategies when the first attempt does not work?

7. Does the student "catch on " to directions quickly or need extra examples or explanation? (May see this more in work evaluation than in standardized testing).

8. Does the student identify the need for clarification and ask? (Know when they don't know) Does the student need constant reassurance (How am I doing?)

9. Are verbal abilities commensurate with "doing" abilities? (Verbal-performance gap?)

10. How predictable was this student? Was performance consistent or highly variable? (Must consider the effect of antecedent information).

11. How fast or slow was this student in processing information and completing tasks and how did this processing style affect performance on various tasks?

■□ ISSUES IN THE TESTING OF ADOLESCENTS.

Those of us working with adolescents question the assumption that language development issues not resolved in elementary school are hopeless. Adolescents must continue to develop language and will often need help as they encounter the challenges of higher-level language tasks. Yvlisaker and DeBonis (2000) suggest that some adolescents can "grow into a disability" when undetected frontal lobe lesions cause interference as cognitive demands increase at transitions to higher level demands. We won't know, of course, if there are actual lesions in those adolescents having difficulty when we "up the ante" as they progress to higher grades in school (Tattershall, 1994b), but we do need to find out how their abilities match the requirements at these times. We need to test their language and learning in order to help adolescents devise appropriate plans for adequate communication and learning at higher levels of school and beyond. This seems clear given the concerns about preventing high school dropouts (Lord-Larson & McKinley, 1995), the high incidence of language and learning problems in prisons and detention centers including 75–90% of juvenile offenders (Newman, Lewis, & Beverstock, 1993) and general concerns about difficulties of youngsters going through adolescence. In view of recent, well publicized violent acts committed in schools, it is clearly appropriate to assess communication and learning abilities as part of our attempts to understand and help adolescents.

Helping Adolescents Accept Testing

It is not always easy to assess adolescents. They do not want to be identified as different from their peers, so testing has to be presented as a natural way to learn about strengths and weaknesses rather than a tool for merely identifying those in serious trouble. Examiners who appreciate that all adolescents have learning strengths and needs; who see those with known labels (ADHD, LD, Language-disordered, etc.) as having skills and/or problems on a continuum with others; who acknowledge that most students will have a profile of multiple intelligences and do not view adolescents with learning problems as an "exotic species" may be able to allay adolescents' concerns simply by the way in which they interact in the testing situation. If everyone in a diagnostic process remembers to identify strengths along with weaknesses, adolescents may be more motivated to participate. Ylvisaker, Feeney and Feeney (1999) discuss the important first step in a functional intervention program that includes finding out "what is working and what is not working." Recognizing strengths initially can keep the adolescent encouraged especially when the strengths can be useful in improving weak areas defined in the diagnostic process and through shoulder-to-shoulder collaboration.

Finding Time for Testing

It is difficult to find time to test adolescents. Taking them out of class can be a problem at the beginning of a school term because classroom routines are being established along with content review and/or development of a common information base for new concepts. Teachers may not appreciate the need for testing language when a student's short conversational exchanges show clear speech and appropriate basic sentence structure. One high school student engaged easily in a short interchange but lost many points on an important term paper grade because he misunderstood the directions, a typical problem for him. Even when many other examples of misunderstandings in conversation and in reading text were provided, the teacher remained unconvinced of a language problem because of this youngster's clear speech and ability to engage in appropriate short interchanges. That teacher might resent releasing this student for testing.

After school activities and part-time employment also make scheduling difficult, but assessment is important enough that we have to be creative in finding time and ways to test effectively. Testing can start the problem solving process.

Considering Intelligence in Assessment

Those working with adolescents with language and learning difficulties want to know their intellectual potential and to consider the possible interaction of language and intellectual ability shown on tests. We need to know how the results of intellectual assessment correlate to actual performance in and out of classrooms. Parents and others working in collaboration with parents are constantly trying to discriminate the "can't versus won't" factor in school performance, that is, how much of an adolescent's problem is related to ability and how much to motivation. Intelligence tests can help us understand what an adolescent's potential might be. Sternberg (1981) described three components of intelligence: being able to profit from experience in order to learn and acquire knowledge, being able to reason effectively, and being able to adapt to changes. Sternberg (1981) also discussed the impact of a student's motivation on development of intelligence. Nelson (1998) discussed the possible impact of economic, social and cultural factors along with communication abilities on intellectual assessment. Testing intelligence is a complicated issue and it is difficult to interpret the results particularly to adolescents who can be dramatically affected by scores that seem to limit their potential. However, intelligence testing is one measure that can inform our problem solving work with adolescents.

The *Wechsler Intelligence Test for Children* (third edition), WISC-III, and the *Wechsler Adult Intelligence Scale* (third edition), WAIS-3, (Wechsler, 1939–1997a & b) are frequently the intelligence tests of choice and can answer questions including the following: "What is the overall intellectual range of ability? Is there a relative strength in verbal ability over performance or vice versa? Does this seem to reflect vocabulary and other language abilities? Is there scatter among subtests and what patterns has the psychologist observed?" The index scores in the third edition include a Verbal Comprehension Index, Perceptual Organization Index, a Working Memory Index and Processing Speed. Hess (1998) reviewed the WAIS-3 and noted three new subtests: Symbol

Search that allows for assessing processing speed, Letter-Number Sequencing that allows for measuring working memory and Matrix Reasoning that allows observation of nonverbal untimed abstract reasoning. This reviewer noted that although there are still timed tasks, the timed aspect has been de-emphasized in the new edition, a factor that might be of help in allowing adolescents with delayed processing or test anxiety to better demonstrate intelligence. A second reviewer, Rogers (1998), reported that the WAIS is the oldest and most frequently used intelligence scale for individual administration to adults but he expressed concern about the pictures in the new test not adequately portraying what they purported to test.

The *Kaufman Adolescent and Adult Intelligence Test*, KAIT (Kaufman & Kaufman, 1993) is intended for those 11 through 85 years of age. The Crystallized Scale measures acquired knowledge and the Fluid Scale measures ability to solve new problems. Their six subtests in the Core Battery include definitions, rebus learning, logical steps, auditory comprehension, mystery codes and double meanings. The Expanded Battery adds four additional subtests.

The *Slosson Intelligence Test–Revised* (Slosson, Nicholson, & Hibpshman, 1990) can be administered to those age 4 through adulthood. This test is considered a quick estimate of general verbal ability. One reviewer, R. W. Kamphaus (1995,) stated a preference for the *Kaufman Brief Intelligence Test*, the K-BIT, (Kaufman & Kaufman, 1990) for "stronger evidence of concurrent validity and a less verbal screener" than that offered by the Slosson. The K-BIT tests those of 4 to 90 years, measures verbal functions including expressive vocabulary and definitions along with nonverbal functions through the matrices subtest purported to measure fluid thinking and ability to solve new problems by perceiving relationships and completing analogies

Using Results from Nonverbal Intelligence Measures

There are nonverbal intelligence tests developed, ostensibly, to minimize verbal demands for those with language problems in order to investigate their language-free intellectual ability. This is a laudable goal but there are problems. Nelson (1998) expressed concern that these measures can give a limited view of nonverbal cognition; that they may demand attention to only physical characteristics of visual stimuli (Johnston, 1982) and can require perceptual rather than a full conceptual processing (Kamhi, Minor, & Mauer, 1990). Nelson observed that because language-disordered children lack the advantage of verbal mediation they may not encode key features of the stimuli. The caution then is to use nonverbal intelligences tests with awareness of their limitations and with informed clinical judgment.

The *Test of Nonverbal Intelligence*—TONI-3, (Brown, Sherbenau & Johnsen, 1997) measures aptitude and reasoning of those from ages 5 through 85–11, does not require oral or written language skill, and can be given in 5–20 minutes. The *Comprehensive Test of Nonverbal Intelligence*,

CTONI (Hammill, Pearson & Wiederholt, 1996) can also be given in a computer administered version (CTONI-CA). This test requires one hour and provides three composite scores: Nonverbal Intelligence Quotient; Pictorial Nonverbal Intelligence Quotient; and Geometric Nonverbal Intelligence Quotient. One reviewer, G. Aylward, (1998), favored the combination of pictorial and geometric context and the absence of purely perceptual measures in this test.

The *Leiter-R*, (Roid & Miller, 1996) can be given to those 2–0 through 20–11. It includes a battery for Visualization and Reasoning that was also in the former test and a new battery, Attention and Memory. There is no reading or writing required and the publishers present the instrument as appropriate for those who are cognitively delayed, disadvantaged, non-verbal, or non-English speakers, or those who have speech, hearing or motor impairments, ADHD, autism or TBI. There are "growth" scores that purport to measure small improvements in those with significant cognitive impairments. There are also rating scales to be completed by parents, teachers, examiners and the adolescent addressing activity level, attention, impulse control and other emotional factors. The test reportedly correlates with the WISC-III at 0.85.

The *Universal Nonverbal Intelligence Test*, UNIT (Bracken & McCallum, 1998) is designed for those 5 years to 17–11, includes an abbreviated and standard form, results in a full-scale quotient, reasoning quotient, memory quotient, symbolic and nonsymbolic quotients. There are multiple response modes including use of manipulatives, paper and pencil and pointing. The publishers suggest that this test is appropriate for those with speech-language and hearing impairments, different culture or language and/or those who are verbally noncommunicative.

The *Stanford-Binet Intelligence Scale, fourth edition, nonverbal short form* (Glaub & Kamphaus, 1991) is designed for use with those of 2 years through 23 years and is composed of five subtests taken from the full fourth edition and requiring the least verbal responses: Bead Memory, Pattern Analysis, Copying, Memory for Objects, and Matrices. This nonverbal short form is intended for the hearing impaired, and those with speech language disorders or limited English.

Putting the Intelligence Scores in Perspective

It has been helpful, in my experience, when the examiner reporting results of an intelligence assessment offers observations about the possible effects of anxiety in test taking, language difficulties, memory problems or other mitigating factors. These observations, along with others contributed through informal measures can help us better understand a student's intellectual functioning and help the adolescent appreciate the need for "integration of background information, behavior observations and other test scores ... " with that of the intellectual assessment results (Kaufman, 1979., p. 9). Schema theory suggests that language, cognition, social and emotional factors affect each other and that their interaction makes it difficult to isolate them for independent study (Highman, 1994). Adolescents need to view intelligence testing results with this in mind.

Considering the Ability–Achievement Discrepancy Model

The ability–achievement discrepancy model uses intelligence testing results as the standard for ability and for comparison with achievement scores in determining learning discrepancies. Siegel (1992) questioned the assumptions underlying the use of IQ in defining learning disabilities suggesting that the correlation between IQ and reading is low, that there is a lack of consensus about the extent of discrepancy between reading achievement and potential estimated by IQ and that the diagnosis of reading disabilities based on IQ may satisfy administrative requirements for student placement but may not lead to recommendations for instruction. Hooper et al., (1994) suggested that rather than using intelligence measures one compare listening comprehension (ability) with reading comprehension (achievement) and, for writing, to observe differences between oral expression and written expression to define specific learning problems. Aaron and Baker (1991) favor the use of listening comprehension in place of IQ to determine reading problems. Berninger, Hart, Abbott and Karovsky (1992) suggested, instead of using IQ as the standard, to use an absolute criterion, an academic deficit that falls significantly below the mean to first identify children in need of intervention. Those identified could then, in these authors' plan, be separated into those with low functioning, underachievement and learning disability with the use of an ability–achievement formula to determine need for special education. Of course the discrepancy formula will show only discrepancy. Observation and trial teaching may be necessary to best understand the reasons for delays. Nelson (1998) has discussed the problems with discrepancy criterion and questioned the assumption that "only children who show a discrepancy need specialized interventions to succeed in school" (p. 97).

Exploring Executive Function

Executive function can be a critical factor in assessing the abilities of youngsters. Denckla (1994) discusses the elements of interference control, effortful and flexible organization, and strategic planning as the undisputed factors in executive function. She notes that working memory and attention are also issues in execution function and advises the considering of attention to the present and future in order to assess ability to plan. Denckla reports that one of the difficulties in testing for executive function is that one must test responses to novel stimuli so a test–retest format cannot be followed. Denckla (1994, p. 124) listed tests used to assess various factors in executive function such as concept formation (*Wisconsin Card Sort Test*, Heaton, Chehine, Talley, Hay, &

Curtiss, 1981–1993); spatial planning, (*Rey-Osterreith Complex Figure*, Meyers & Meyers, 1995); memorizing (*California Verbal Learning Test*, Delis et al., 1994; 2000); inhibiting, speed efficiency, interference control, visual detail (*Matching Familiar Figures Test*); semantic strategy (*20 Questions*). Executive function seems an important area to consider for many adolescents who have adequate individual skills as tested but cannot "put it together" for effective performance in school or on the job.

Learning Aptitude, Information Processing, and Memory

The *Detroit Tests of Learning Aptitude-Adult* (Hammill & Bryant, 1991) are designed to show intelligence, aptitude and achievement and to identify those adults with "markedly deficient" general mental ability. These tests include twelve subtests and eight composite scores including Linguistic Verbal and Nonverbal; Attention Enhanced and Reduced; Motor Enhanced and Reduced, General Mental Ability and Optimal.

The *Detroit Test of Learning Aptitude*, fourth edition (DTLA-4), is designed for those 6 years through 17 years (Hammill & Bryant, 1991), has ten subtests, and provides an overall composite score; an optimal level composite composed of the four highest standard scores presumably showing optimal potential and contrasting composites for language, attention and manual dexterity.

The *Ross Information Processing Assessment*, second edition (RIPA-2) (Ross-Swain, 1996) for ages 15 through 90 assesses immediate and recent memory, temporal orientation, spatial orientation, orientation to environment, recall of general information, problem solving and abstract reasoning, organization and auditory processing and retention. This tests purports to distinguish between those with cognitive deficits and those with normal cognitive skills.

The *Test of Memory and Learning* (TOMAL) (Reynolds & Bigler, 1994) for ages 5–19 includes assessment of Verbal Memory, Nonverbal Memory, Delayed Recall, and Composite Memory Index; Learning Index, Attention and Concentration Index; Sequential Memory Index; Free Recall Index; and Associate Recall Index.

Many tests sample memory for digits, sentence repetition and/or require that those taking the test keep items in memory in order to do something else, and we need to keep memory issues in our own minds as test givers or data users. For instance, many of the subtests on the *Clinical Evaluation of Language Fundamentals*, third edition, and other tests do not allow the stimulus sentences or words be repeated. The Word Classes subtest asks students to hold three or four words in mind in order to identify two words that go together. The score from this test can mean that the student does not understand the relationships among words or that he or she cannot remember them. So whether one is investigating memory directly or not, it is an issue in many tests.

Checking Perceptual Motor Abilities

Testing of hearing, vision and motor abilities helps guide planning for adolescents. Results of peripheral hearing tests combined with the history of middle ear infections, P.E. tubes, allergies, upper respiratory infections, tonsillectomy and adenoidectomy are important for their possible contributions to the students' processing of information. If there is a known hearing loss, we need to know when it was detected, the pattern and severity of the loss, if amplification has been used and when it was first obtained, if the adolescent has worn the aids consistently and continues to wear aids and/or to use amplification in the classroom along with other accommodations.

Considering Auditory Processing

Discussions of auditory processing abilities provoke different opinions. There are those who feel there is an identifiable group whose primary difficulties involve auditory processing. There are others who feel that this group is not so clearly defined and that the issue is one of comprehension or processing of language rather than a specific central auditory processing disorder. Nelson (1998) discussed the research of Tallal and her associates (Tallal, 1980; Tallal & Piercy, 1978; Tallal & Stark, 1976) that suggested a generalized sequential processing defect for rapid auditory and visual stimuli and that children with language learning impairments presented symptoms reflecting "bottom up processing constraints rather than a defect in language competence per se" (Tallal et al., 1996, p. 6). Nelson cited another study that failed to show significant differences in brain stem responses to acoustic tone shifts in children with specific language impairment (Tomblin, Abbas, Records, & Brenneman, 1995). Nelson questioned whether a defect in the central auditory processing mechanism causes or reflects a language system that is not working effectively.

Various professionals interpret the information from testing of central auditory processing ability differently, but the results can be helpful. In my work with adolescents, the term "auditory processing disorder" seems to describe problems that result from a variety of causes including language difficulties, inconsistent or poor attention often caused by limited understanding of various scripts and contexts for communication, differences in arousal often attached to interest or differences in the level of language that attracts those with various attention styles. The information from auditory processing testing can guide observations and planning with students by showing whether the student has difficulty attending to sound in noise, for example, which leads to identifying situations where this might be an issue and devising strategies or plans for those situations. The suggestions made after central auditory processing testing can be helpful for many children and adolescents with listening or attention problems.

A checklist of common features of central auditory processing disorders (CAPD) can help specify problems and lead to plans. Such a list provided by Paton (Internet article reprint, 2001) includes the following features to describe problems of a person with CAPD:

1. Talks or likes TV louder than normal.
2. Interprets words too literally.
3. Often needs remarks repeated; gets important messages wrong.
4. Difficulty sounding out words.
5. "Ignores" people, especially if engrossed.
6. Unusually sensitive to sounds.
7. Asks many extra-informational questions.
8. Confuses similar-sounding words.
9. Difficulty following directions in a series or forgets instructions; makes "silly" mistakes or "careless" errors caused by intrusions of random sounds that break concentration.
10. Speech developed late or unclearly.
11. Poor "communicator" (terse, telegraphic); difficulty knowing "what to say when" caused by difficulty noting tonality of the voice.
12. Memorizes poorly.
13. Hears better when watching the speaker; has trouble hearing clearly in a noisy place; misses important sounds and signals.
14. Problems with rapid speech.

This list seems to include effects of listeners not knowing the context of the conversation or being inattentive to intraword differences, perhaps because of a focus on meaning rather than form; of listeners being bottom line communicators who are overly economical in their own comments, do not appreciate another speaker's need for elaboration and "tune out" when information seems redundant; of those who need to be very sure about information and become overloaded when information comes in too quickly—evidence of various communication styles. Whether one views these as central auditory defects causing communication differences, characteristics reflecting language disorders or evidence of varying attention styles, the list can help specify problems interfering with language processing in learning.

The *SCAN-A*, test for auditory processing disorders–adolescents and adults (Keith,1994), includes subtests for filtered words, auditory figure ground, competing words and competing sentences. The *Goldman-Fristoe-Woodcock Auditory Skills Test Battery* (Goldman, Fristoe, & Woodcock, 1976) is designed for use with those of 3 years through adult for testing of auditory selective attention, diagnostic auditory discrimination, auditory memory and sound–symbol associations. The *Goldman-Fristoe-Woodcock Test of Auditory Discrimination* (Goldman, Fristoe, & Woodcock, 1970). is intended for those from 3 years 8 months through 70 years and tests for word discrimination in quiet and in noise. The AGS manual explains that this test is "geared to young children's vocabulary levels" (p. 5) suggesting that it may not be appropriate for adolescents with age-appropriate vocabulary knowledge.

Barkley (1994) in discussing measures for attention reported that children with ADHD have more difficulty with sustained attention than with focus or selective attention (disengage, move, engage), a factor to consider when reviewing testing. Of course, one must consider that those with ADHD can also have language problems that can cause difficulty in focusing on the pertinent aspect when asked to sort out meaning. The "wheat from chaff" (Chapter 7) principle may be a problem for some adolescents who also have difficulty with sustained attention. In other words they may not know what is most important and they may not be able to concentrate long enough to figure it out.

Listening and Attention

It is difficult to separate listening from that included in assessment of language processing, receptive language tasks, central auditory processing, and so forth. The context in which listening occurs seems so important along with the topic, motivation and background information, that assessing listening by itself seems contrived. There are measures that focus on listening; and, we can probably learn something from observing students within these tasks if our observations are supported by those in a variety of situations.

There are listening components within the *TOAL-3* and the *CELF-3*. The *Diagnostic Reading Scales* (Spache, 1995) have parallel forms for listening and reading comprehension. The *Stanford Achievement Test: Listening Comprehension Tests* (Harcourt Brace, 1992a) apparently ask students to listen to very complex, dense language perhaps more appropriate for reading and reflecting than listening. A reading comprehension measure that includes two forms, such as the Passage Comprehension subtest of the *Woodcock Reading Mastery Tests, Revised* (Forms G & H) can be used informally to compare comprehension in listening and reading, with the understanding that this is a comparison of written language in two modalities. It seems critical, in any case, to view listening within the context in which it should occur. Adolescents who do not show difficulty on competing auditory signals in central auditory testing, for instance, may not be skilled at attending to instructors and at the same time monitoring what is going on socially with their classmates. This is a listening problem that may reflect their not knowing body language or other social cues automatically. They need to be more vigilant than those who can listen to the teacher effectively while also keeping their social antennae ready for something pertinent that may require their response.

Some instruments that can be used with adolescents to assess attention include the *Brief Test of Attention* (Schretian, 1997) which is an auditory perception task providing assessment of attention in the verbal–linguistic system. It is designed for adults with visual and motor impairments and does not require visual scanning or manual dexterity. It is standardized for ages 17 to 82 years and has two forms presented on audiocassette. The *Attention-Deficit/Hyperactivy Disorder Test*, ADHDT, (Gilliam, 1995) is a norm referenced behavior rating checklist based on the DSM-IV. There are 3 subtests: hyperactivity, impulsivity, and inattention. This test can be administered by parents, teachers or others for ages 3–23.

Considering Vision

Vision screening is, of course, important in our understanding and helping adolescents. We need to know if adolescents can see adequately, what kind of visual problems they may have, when they were identified and what kind of help they have received. Just as we need to know when hearing aids were prescribed, how consistently the adolescent wears the aids, and if not/why not, we need to answer these same questions about glasses. Diagnostic measures for visual function beyond acuity have been controversial. There are professionals and parents who strongly recommend the testing of visual function, and feel that subsequent visual remediation measures are necessary and helpful in facilitating effective learning. Vellutino (1979b) suggested through his research that visual perception is not the usual culprit in dyslexia and that reading is a language based activity rather than being dependent primarily on vision. I have participated in diagnostic teams with an optometrist who is a passionate advocate of vision training. As a professional who views issues through the lens of language development and use, I often differ with his interpretation of behavior, but I also learn from his observations and have a broader view of the adolescent in question. In any case, I feel that it is important to know if and how the adolescent hears and sees; what observations have been made; and to use these findings along with other information to understand and help adolescents.

Learning about Coordination, Movement, Position in Space

Occupational and physical therapy testing is not always available or even necessary for all adolescents but there are many times when this information is desirable. For those adolescents who have a difficult time finding their social place with peers, for instance, I wonder if they are grounded in space, that is, if they know where they are in relation to the chair, the floor, the ceiling, and so forth. Are they so preoccupied with maintaining themselves in space that they don't notice the nonverbal cues of others, for example? I think of adolescents with pragmatic language problems and wonder if their orientation in space might be contributing to their difficulties. Perhaps early identification of sensorimotor competence with subsequent intervention might have established a base for appropriate attention and language development. I am reminded of two very bright adolescent boys, for instance, who struggled socially in spite of academic success. One boy was so uncoordinated that his friends teased him constantly about the time he "almost hung himself trying to lower the shade so we could watch a movie in class." This same young man seemed to lecture others rather than engage in a conversation, rarely looking at his listener to monitor understanding, agreement or their need for a conversational turn. The second young man was somewhat clumsy and overbearing, often alienating peers with his bragging. Both students could read fluently in kindergarten but were described as "clumsy" and "immature" causing their teachers to recommend a second year in kindergarten. An occupational therapy assessment might have shown problems and guided planning in ways that other information did not.

Another adolescent with selective mutism presented with an unusual lumbering gait with toes turned inward in a "pigeon toed" fashion. He seemed to lean forward with his upper body as though he were always walking into a hard wind. In addition, this sweet natured, very tall young man wore a constant scowl exaggerated by a heavy crease above his eyebrows. The effect of his physical movement, expression and silence was often frightening, exacerbating his social interactional problems. The insight of physical and occupational therapists seemed an important element in helping this young man.

Investigating Oral Language

When we consider adolescents' oral language, we need to know about vocabulary knowledge as it affects language processing. We need to know about word retrieval, about sentence level competence and about adolescents' ability to manage longer discourse—beyond sentences. We need to know about the appropriateness of adolescents' communication and their speech clarity. We need to check their ability to listen effectively in a variety of settings and to determine how various settings affect listening, to note how intellectual abilities, language abilities and individual learning style and/or personality affect listening. We need to know how effectively adolescents identify and express their need for clarification. Do they notice when problems occur in listening? How do they react when they do not understand? Are there culture-based customs that inhibit asking questions, particularly of superiors? Do they "read" body language and the situation in order to gain information? We need to investigate the strengths and weaknesses adolescents present for taking in information.

Testing for Vocabulary Knowledge

The *Peabody Picture Vocabulary Test*, third edition (PPVT-III) (Dunn & Dunn, 1997) is described as useful for screening verbal ability, giftedness, mental retardation, and English language proficiency along with detecting language impairments, and so forth. (p. 3, examiner's manual). The manual suggests that the PPVT-III can serve as "one element in a comprehensive test battery of cognitive processes" when English is the native language spoken at home. In practice, the PPVT-III is typically used to assess receptive, single word knowledge. It is often the first formal test in my typical diagnostic routine and allows for observation of the adolescent's style in test taking including risk taking, impulsiveness, and so forth. It is also, as suggested in the manual (p. 3), useful in establishing rapport because it does not require oral responses and does not seem threatening. The results of this test and others tapping vocabulary knowledge contribute to the understanding of the adolescents' world experience associated with vocabulary and suggest something about attention style. For instance, some students seem to have had extensive opportunities and stimulation provided by middle-class, educated parents but have apparently not noticed or retained new vocabulary reflecting that experience. There are other adolescents who have admittedly read very little but have surprisingly good receptive vocabulary knowledge, suggesting a strength in learning through listening. The results from the *Peabody* can sometimes explain sight word reading ability. For instance, students with limited phonologic abilities but good receptive vocabulary knowledge can sometimes recognize words they cannot spell and lack skills for decoding unfamiliar words in reading. Those with low scores on the *PPVT-3* might also have low sight word identification scores in reading because they are simultaneously trying to read and learn new vocabulary. This relatively simple picture identification task and other receptive vocabulary tests described below can be helpful in knowing adolescents.

The *Expressive Vocabulary Test* (EVT) (Williams, 1997), for ages 2–6 through 90+ years was standardized on the same population as the *PPVT-III* allowing direct comparisons in receptive and expressive vocabulary on these measures.

The *Comprehensive Receptive and Expressive Vocabulary Tests* (CREVT) is also available in a computer administered format (CREVT-CA) for ages 4 through 17 years 11 months (Wallace & Hammill, 1994; 1997). The format for the receptive portion of the test includes pictures grouped by theme. The *Comprehensive Receptive and Expressive Vocabulary Test–Adult* (CREVT-A) addresses ages 18–0 through 89–11 (1997).

The *Receptive One Word Picture Vocabulary Test 2000* (ROWPVT-2000) and the *Expressive One Word Picture Vocabulary Test 2000* (EOW-PVT-2000) (Brownell, 2000a; 2000b) have been co-normed so that comparisons can be made between receptive and expressive vocabulary scores for 2 years through 18 years 11 months.

The *WORD* test–Adolescent (Zachman, Huisingh, Barrett, Orman, & Blagden, 1989) assesses expressive vocabulary and semantic knowledge for 12–17 year olds with subtests asking for explanations of brand names, for synonyms, for interpretation of signs, and for definitions.

The *Test of Adolescent/Adult Word Finding* (TAWF) (German, 1990) for ages 12–80 and grades 7–12, assesses accuracy and speed in picture naming of nouns and verbs; in sentence completion, in description and in category naming. A comprehension section is included to help distinguish word finding from comprehension. The normative data address response time and there is also an informal analysis of gestures, extra-verbalization and substitution types.

Other Language Tests

The *Test of Adolescent and Adult Language*, third edition (TOAL-III) (Hammill, Brown, Larsen & Wiederholt, 1994) is designed to assess the linguistic aspects of listening, speaking, reading and writing. There are eight subtests and composite quotients for total language, reading, writing, speaking, spoken language and written language, vocabulary and grammar, receptive and expressive language. The vocabulary subtests on the *Test of Adolescent and Adult Language*, third edition, tap knowledge of multiple meanings, ability to make sentences with given words along with ability to identify words in categories providing a more complete understanding of the students' word knowledge in listening, reading and writing tasks to add to their recognition vocabulary shown by the *PPVT-3*. Speaking Vocabulary and Writing Vocabulary, the sentence making tasks on the TOAL-III, are considered expressive measures on this test, but they contribute information about vocabulary knowledge that affects understanding. The sentence combining task, Writing Grammar, elicits complex sentences but there is no extended discourse required in any of the subtests.

The *Clinical Evaluation of Language Fundamentals*, third edition (CELF-III) (Semel, Wiig, & Secord, 1994) has norms extended to 21 years 11 months and can be used with adolescents. There are three receptive subtests (Concepts and Directions, Word Classes, Semantic Relationships) along with a supplementary subtest (Listening to Paragraphs). I have found it interesting to use the Listening to Paragraphs both in its intended form and, informally, as a reading comprehension task. The three expressive tasks (Formulated Sentences, Recalling Sentences and Sentence Assembly) focus on sentence level knowledge in somewhat contrived formats. Verification using language sampling within various conversations and/or for school language purposes seems required to check real world sentence making. Although the CELF-III is regularly used for school-aged youngsters, the TOAL-III seems to offer challenges more consistent with upper level classrooms and to be my choice for students at 8th grade level and above, although the focus is still on sentences more than discourse in both tests.

The *Adolescent Language Screening Test* (ALST) (Morgan & Guilford, 1984) allows for rapid screening of pragmatics, receptive vocabulary, concepts, expressive vocabulary, sentence formulation, morphology and phonology.

The *Fullerton Language Test for Adolescents*, second edition (Thorum, 1986) measures receptive and expressive language for those from 11 years through adult. There are eight subtests including Auditory Synthesis, Morphology Competency, Oral Commands, Convergent

Production, Divergent Production, Syllabication, Grammatic Competency and Idioms.

The *Test of Language Competence,* expanded version (TLC-E) (Wiig & Secord, 1989), level 2 is designed for those from 9–0 to 18–0 years and purports to assess metalinguistic competence and linguistic strategies for semantics, syntax, and/or pragmatics. The subtests that tap receptive abilities, "interpreting intents" show students' ability to make inferences and to understand figurative expressions. The remaining subtests, although billed as "expressing intents" seem to require understanding of ambiguity and appreciation of situations and intent in order to create sentences from several words. This test provides contexts for tasks that help one to observe students' world experience and understanding in context. There is a contrived quality about the tasks but this distance from real world interaction can show exactly what the tests are designed to assess, that is the ability to reflect consciously on language meaning. The TLC-E can offer insights that can be verified in or contrasted with actual communication. I can envision, for example, a youngster who has appropriate pragmatic skills in real world interactions but does not have the metalinguistic ability to show this unconscious ability—one who makes a poor test score but might be able to converse adequately.

Evaluating Communicative Competence (ECC) (Simon, 1986) is a functional pragmatic procedure for students 9–17 years. It is an informal measure that results in a description of communication ability, but strives for objectivity by asking the examiner to provide percentages for performances. The test is lengthy and demanding to administer and may be more practical to give in diagnostic therapy than in initial one session testing, but it can provide rich information about receptive and expressive language.

The *Modern Language Aptitude test* (MLAT) (Carroll & Sapon, 1959) has been discussed for its part in determining the inclusion of students with learning disability in a modified foreign language class in college. Downey and Snyder (2000) suggested that appropriate placement in such a class requires an MLAT score lower than the 10th percentile and that the student score at least 1 standard deviation below the mean on reading and spelling on the *Wide Range Achievement Test* (Wilkinson, 1994).

Assessing Articulation and Phonologic Ability

There are a variety of tests of articulation that include adolescents and adults but for the most part, the pictures do not seem appropriate for this age group. For instance, the *Goldman-Fristoe Test of Articulation,* second edition (2000) lists an age range of 2–21 years but one catalog included the comment that the "duck is even cuter" in the new edition confirming the impression that the pictures are made to appeal to young children. Other articulation measures with adolescent age ranges include the *Comprehensive Articulation Test* (Weiss, 1980); the *Fisher-Logemann Test of Articulation Competence* (Fisher & Logemann,

1971) P–adult. For many adults it is practical for an experienced speech language pathologist to assess articulation in conversation and/or during oral reading testing. Sight word reading measures often allow for close observation of sound production, for instance. For the severely unintelligible adult, the use of pictures and/or reading of single words from the articulation tests may be necessary.

The *Comprehensive Test of Phonological Processing* (Wagner, Torgesen, & Rashotte, 1999) covers ages 5–0 through 24–11. It assesses phonologic awareness, phonologic memory and rapid naming. The subtests include Elision, Blending Words, Sound Matching, Memory for Digits, Nonword Repetition, Rapid Color Naming, Rapid Digit Naming, Rapid Letter Naming, Rapid Object Naming, Blending Nonwords, Phoneme Reversal, Segmenting Words and Segmenting Nonwords.

The *Lindamood Auditory Conceptualization Test* (LAC) (Lindamood & Lindamood, 1979) for all ages measures discrimination of phonemes and segmentation of words into constituent phonemes.

We need to know how well adolescents understand others and express their own ideas in a variety of situations: in conversations, in whole classroom discussions, in small groups for short interchanges requiring clear speech and basic sentence structure as compared with situations requiring organized lengthy discourse. We need to know about their pragmatic skills. For example, are they expressing themselves appropriately, reflecting their appreciation of their listener and the various roles of participants, as well as the requirements of the setting? We need to know how students manage both oral and written language

Exploring Written Language

In order to work productively with adolescents and to predict the difficulty they might have in school, we need to know about their reading ability. We need to know about the level, automaticity and accuracy of single word reading and compare this information to oral vocabulary knowledge and phonologic awareness evidenced in oral language and spelling. We need to know about ability to read orally. Reading assessments sometimes focus on silent reading for adolescents; however, many students live in fear of embarrassing themselves if called upon to read aloud. So we need to know about oral reading in order to help ("How do you feel about reading aloud in class? What exactly bothers you about it? Are you afraid you might 'mess up'? Do you feel that you read too fast or too slowly?"). We need to know about oral reading fluency, if there is hesitation before content words suggesting a "hangover" from earlier difficulty in word decoding, if reading is too rapid with a racing quality that does not reflect active processing of meaning, if the reader reads in a rhythmic pattern pausing after two or three words regardless of meaning. We need to know if adolescents' reading signals adequate "comprehend*ing*" or monitoring at the sentence level of language as evidenced by miscues resulting in good sentences. We need to compare this sentence level reading with the ability to retell what is read showing "comprehen*sion*" of longer discourse (Weaver, 1980, p. 182). This comprehending–comprehension distinction can identify the level of language focus and competence in adolescents' reading. Many students can read basic sentences but cannot connect meanings and organize them into longer discourse. Others seem to keep track of the thread running through the story and to stay abreast of the theme but to miss supporting detail. We need to know what kinds of reading miscues are made. For example: Do the miscues preserve meaning and good sentence form? Do they look like and sound like the overall word? Do they share only the first sound or syllable of the target word? Are miscues noted and self-corrected by the student or do they simply read on? An informal reading miscue inventory (Goodman & Burke, 1972; Weaver, 1994) in which miscues are analyzed to reveal language strategies in reading and can make the standardized scores meaningful. The *Basic Reading Inventory*, seventh edition (Johns, 1997) provides reading passages through 12th grade level for determining the level of oral reading (independent, instructional, frustrational) based on the total number of miscues and the number of "significant" miscues, that is, miscues that do not change meaning. The comprehension level can also be determined from the retelling and answers to questions. This process is not as thorough as the reading miscue inventory but is a practical compromise that results in levels for comparison and a measure of quality of reading.

We need to know about students' comprehension of different kinds of reading material. To assess comprehension, we can use cloze procedures and paraphrasing of sentences to check sentence level comprehension (Can the student select a word for the blank showing use of word order and grammatical correctness? Can the student restate the sentence in his/her own words and retain the meaning?) We can request retelling of paragraphs and longer sections to check discourse level comprehension. (Can the student accurately identify the topic, main idea and supporting information?) We can note adolescents' attention to and use of cohesive markers to connect meanings over phrase and sentence boundaries. ("Notice the pointing words, 'this, these, those,' what do they mean? What are they pointing back to?").

Having trained oneself to attend to these aspects of reading within informal measures one begins to also notice them within formal testing. In a standardized word reading task, for instance, if the miscues are written by the examiner along with the required correct–incorrect indication, one can notice if oral vocabulary limitations or strengths seem reflected in reading words and/or how reading miscues correspond to the adolescent's spelling attempts or oral pronunciations. In a standardized connected reading task, one can observe pauses that indicate how the reader is attending to thoughts within sentences. One can gain information about a student's natural language focus and ability for sound, word, sentence and short passage levels. One can observe the students' awareness of difficulty as the passages lengthen and how this affects their responses. Some students give up as soon as they see longer sentences. Others persist until the number of difficult words makes it impossible to use context to support their word reading problems. Some students can explain how they knew a passage would be difficult and others cannot, even though they clearly pause before difficult words or sigh when a passage seems long suggesting limited metalinguistic ability. Some students persist in trying when it seems more appropriate to acknowledge that passages are becoming too difficult. These observations (see Box 6–2) can make standardized testing

---

BOX 6–2: *Informal Diagnostic Questions Useful in Formal Reading Testing*

- How automatic is word reading ability in oral reading?
- How does the reader's oral vocabulary knowledge compare with single word reading?
- How fluent is connected oral reading? Are phrasing and pausing appropriate?
- Does the reader pause before content words even when he/she can read them?
- Does the reader show active processing by pausing appropriately for punctuation and/or by breaking up long sentences into thought units?
- Do miscues result in good sentences? Do they fit with the overall passage?
- Do miscues reflect attention to visual aspects of the word: length, overall configuration?
- How does comprehend*ing* (use sentence sense) compare with comprehen*sion* (apparent understanding of the main idea or theme)?
- Can the reader recognize a word within his/her known vocabulary when a word decoding attempt is close to the target word? Or must the attempt be exact to make the closure?
- Is there "head tracking" suggesting a word level focus as during reading?
- In word reading attempts does the reader neglect middle syllables?
- Can they answer fact, inference and opinion questions based on the text?
- Does this reader surprise you by being able to tell the gist of the piece in spite of multiple miscues?
- What happens when the reader encounters a difficult word? Does the reader seem to acknowledge the difficulty or simply slur over and continue on?
- What level of language seems to reflect the reader's focus and/or competence: discourse? sentence? word?

valuable for identifying problems and making plans. Observing formal test taking with a diagnostic ear and eye will yield not just a score, but also qualitative observations to make scores more meaningful. One will be using the test effectively.

Assessing Reading with Formal Tests

There are various categories of norm referenced reading tests: survey tests, diagnostic reading tests, achievement tests, and hybrids of these types.

Survey tests are used to "screen large numbers of students for approximate reading levels and to identify those with severe prob-lems." (Gillet & Temple, 1986) They typically have few subtests and can overestimate reading ability rather than reflect the instructional level in the grade level obtained. They are often formatted as multiple-choice tasks that enable guessing. Survey tests seem to be more effective with average readers than with those at the high or low end of an ability continuum. Some typical survey reading tests include the *Gates-MacGinitie Reading Tests*, third edition (Maginitie & Maginitie, 1989), *Metropolitan Reading Tests*, seventh edition (MA T7) (Harcourt Brace, 1992b) and reading sections of the *Comprehensive Test of Basic Skills*, fourth edition, level 17/18 (CTB/Macmillan, 1989) and *the California Achievement Test*, fifth edition, level K (CTB/McGraw-Hill, 1993).

Diagnostic tests usually include a larger number of subtests and/or test items devised to measure specific skills and the difficulty level tends to be lower allowing for observation of differences among those with reading problems. The *Stanford Diagnostic Reading Test*, fourth edition (SDRT4) (Karlsen & Gardner, 1995) assesses decoding, vocabulary, comprehension and scanning. It assesses fluency for the last three areas mentioned. The *Slosson Oral Reading Test*, revised (Nicholson, 1990) looks only at word recognition with no context as does the reading section of the WRAT-3. The *Gray Oral Reading Test-3* (GORT-3) (Wiederholt & Bryant, 1992) presents words in context allow-ing for observation of oral reading fluency and accuracy. Comprehen-sion questions are asked but are not directly assessed; however, the *Gray Silent Reading Tests* (Wiederholt & Blalock, 2000) for those 7 years through 25 years, presents developmentally sequenced passages each with five multiple choice questions and can be used with the GORT-3.

There are standardized Individual Reading Inventories including the *Durrell Analysis of Reading Difficulty*, third edition (Durrell & Cat-terson, 1980), *Diagnostic Reading Scales* by Spache (1995), *Silvaroli's Classroom Reading Inventory* and the *Ekwall Reading Inventory* which allow for sight word analysis in isolation and in context, silent and oral reading comprehension but there is no qualitative analysis to show types of errors or strategies reflecting a reader's schema about the process. On the Spache, the independent level equals the highest grade level a child can read silently with adequate comprehension and the instructional level is that just below where oral reading breaks down either in word recognition or comprehension. The *Woodcock Reading Mastery Tests*, revised-NU (WRMT-R/NU) (Woodcock, 1987; 1999) provide observations of the reading of real words and nonsense words. These tasks show automatic sight word recall and, if one looks closely at syllable and sound level agreement between miscues and target words, shows phonologic awareness sometimes reflected in and consistent with slurred oral pronunciations of challenging multisyllabic words or those with tongue tip consonants (th, s-z, t-d). The comprehension level subtests tap vocabulary knowledge and thinking (antonyms, synonyms, analogies) as well as ability to select words within cloze passages to show use of sentence and passage level context. The Passage Comprehension subtest from the WRMT-R/NU, a fill-in-the blank task has short passages that do not replicate the length and complexity of typical adolescent curricular materials. This test does not include other comprehension measures such as question answering, a common reading task in classrooms. Students can read the passages silently so information about reading strategies is sometimes lost. Many adolescents begin reading silently, then subvocalize, begin to whisper and finally read aloud in a quiet voice suggesting their need to read orally to better process the information and/or a lack of automaticity or internalizing of skills. Many continue to read silently but move their head from left to right as they read often nodding for each word showing a focus on words rather than phrases. There are others who read silently moving their eyes only without head tracking, the expected mode for an adolescent reader. It is important to appreciate that two readers can achieve the same score on a standardized measure in spite of their using two very different approaches to the task.

The *Test of Word Reading Efficiency* (Wagner, Torgesen & Rashotee, 1999) for those of 6 years through 24–11 measures the number of familiar sight words identified within 45 seconds and the number of non-words accurately decoded within 45 seconds.

The *Nelson-Denny Reading Test*, forms G and H, (Brown, Fishco, & Hanna, 1993) assesses vocabulary, comprehension and reading rate for grades 9–16 and adults and includes separate norms for an extended time condition. The test reportedly predicts academic success, identifies those in need of a developmental reading program or advanced placement, and ranks students in terms of vocabulary, comprehension and reading rate. Reviewers noted little empirical evidence for the ranking, the texts limited to narratives and readability levels of passages were not given (Murray-Ward, 1998; Smith, 1998), but suggested that the concise and practical nature of the test make it appropriate for screening.

The *College Assessment of Academic Progress* (American College Testing, 1996) for ages 17 plus may be used with persons with visual, physical, hearing and mental disabilities and includes a reading test, writing essay test, and writing skills test.

The *Test of Reading Comprehension* (TORC-3) (Brown, Hammill, & Wiederholt, 1995) 7–0 through 17 years 11 months focuses on holistic, cognitive, and linguistic aspects of reading. General reading includes subtests tapping general vocabulary, syntactic similarities, paragraph reading, and sentence sequencing. Diagnostic supplement subtests include measures of content area vocabulary and reading of written directions for schoolwork.

The *Educational Testing Service Test of Applied Literacy Skills for Adults* (1991) assesses document literacy, prose literacy and quantitative literacy in the contexts of workplace, home and community. The test is described as "all open ended, interesting and not intimidating" with an attempt to simulate real world situations. A reviewer (Richards, 1998) noted that the test was well constructed and adaptable to individual clients, that the resulting profile differentiates among different kinds of literacy needed in the workplace, and that there is objective scoring but the scoring and interpretation are elaborate and complex.

Achievement tests are a third type of reading test that include reading as part of a larger battery of tests. A selection of achievement tests can include the *Kaufman Test of Educational Achievement, comprehensive form* (Kaufman & Kaufman, 1985, renormed in 1997) which assesses reading decoding, comprehension along with math and spelling and the *Peabody Individual Achievement Test,* revised (AGS, 1989) which provides assessment in six content areas for those in preschool through post high school. Achievement tests given in schools can be viewed as screening measures that help school systems identify students who fall below expected levels. (Salvia & Ysseldyke, 1991). The *Woodcock-Johnson Pscycho-Educational Battery,* revised—Tests of Achievement, Standard Battery and Supplemental Battery (Woodcock & Johnson, 1990) measure cognitive abilities, scholastic aptitudes and achievement. Age range covers 2 through 90. Both batteries measure reading, mathematics, written language and knowledge.

There are also criterion referenced tests with predetermined instructional outcomes which can result in shaping classrooms to those outcomes, that is, teaching to the test without really assessing reading. These tests can include only the molecular level of reading which is easiest to score but may not replicate the desired reading process. There is also the consideration with these and other tests that some skills may need to be more thoroughly acquired than others within a hierarchy of skills and one cannot know the consistency of performance with one test.

Assessing Writing

Hooper et al. (1994) discussed the need for a writing assessment to take into account endogenous variables: neuropsychologic functions, social-emotional characteristics, and exogenous variables: family functioning, socioeconomic issues, classroom/teaching issues. They also asserted that one must consider as a guide for assessment the characteristics of good writers. Good writers show understanding of the goals in a writing assignment, of the topic and of the intended audience, write more than those who are less proficient, produce more interesting writing with more coherence than that of less proficient writers. Good writers also revise for meaning more than for form at early stages of the writing process. Competent writers of stories include an initiating event showing a problem, attempt to solve, and direct consequence or result. Optional characteristics can include a setting statement to show locations, internal response of characters, and reaction to the outcomes. Finally, these authors stressed the need to consider writing pieces involving imagination, recollection, notation in terms of listing, those requiring "cogitation" such as essays, and those requiring investigation and fact gathering. (Moffett, 1986). A second category to be considered for writing assessment included 1) narration/description; 2) procedural compositions, 3) time-order rendering of events including problem solution or cause/effect and 4) topic exposition requiring argument and supporting detail (Howie, 1984). D'Angelo (1984) provided a list of five types of writing including expressive, narrative, descriptive, expository and argumentative prose as the basics with addition of poetry and drama to the list.

Decisions about how to assess writing include the kinds of writing to be assessed and how to elicit the writing samples. If picture prompts are used they should include 1) at least two characters, 2) an interesting or novel scene, and 3) some kind of potential conflict suggesting and eliciting a sequence of events. (Hooper et al., 1994) The type of prompt can result in varied quality of responses. Prompts can be personalized or neutral in their meaning and therefore elicit a different writing sample (Brossell & Ash, 1984). They can have high or low structural demands, or be long or short with different effects. (Greenberg, 1981; Hoetker & Brossell, 1989).

There is also a list of production components to be considered in evaluating a writer's process. The thinking phase of writing should be observed (generating and organizing ideas and setting goals) followed by translating thinking into written form (making good sentences with appropriate vocabulary spelled correctly with needed punctuation), and the reviewing/revising phase (checking for sense with the audience in mind and for form). We must consider the fluency with which writers manage, think and write revealing underlying skills (brainstorming, grammar, punctuation, spelling) and the ability to produce a coherent passage with old/new information balanced appropriately for the intended reader. The timed versus untimed writing condition must be considered for its effect on writing. There are those who need more time to plan but then write in a timely manner. There can be other writers who produce bursts of ideas quickly but need intermittent pauses for regrouping their thoughts. There are writers who produce clear or beautiful passages but cannot organize their ideas into longer pieces. The environment is also an issue in that some writers need solitude and others can block out distraction.

The *Test of Written Language*, third edition (Hammill & Larsen, 1996). Ages 7–6 through 17 years 11 months provides one way to look at adolescents' writing (through age 17 years 11 months) and to derive standard scores. It seems practical to administer the Spontaneous Writing portion as a screening measure of writing ability but the Contrived Writing tasks seem less helpful in my experience except to show what youngsters can do when focused on parts of the writing task. Observing adolescents writing in response to a picture on the spontaneous writing subtest allows a score for comparison with peers, the opportunity to note if the youngsters begin writing in a timely manner, if they generate ideas fluently, or not, with a stimulus picture, whether they seem to plan and to produce a well-formed story, to elaborate and expand ideas within the time constraints. The resulting writing sample, of course, must be considered along with other samples elicited in a variety of ways to appreciate what is typical writing for the adolescent, how the genre affects the writing, if the timed condition caused a variation from the typical writing, and so on. One needs to know how well adolescents can generate and write about topics of their own, for instance, and if they can refine an assigned general topic to a workable topic. It is important to know whether the students' writing includes a main idea or simply a list of relatively equal ideas, if they can organize both narrative and expository writing, if they can answer essay questions efficiently and effectively, if their writing includes appropriate complexity and expansion of ideas.

Adolescents with language disorders can often produce an adequate but very short, simple piece that looks "young" rather than "wrong." These students do not produce the level of complexity and elaboration of their more successful peers. They may always write in a conversational style without adopting a different style for more formal writing. They may understand the information they want to communicate but be unable to organize their facts appropriately into various forms of discourse. Even their sentence level abilities can be undeveloped with persistent difficulty in noun-verb agreement or appreciation of the difference between a phrase or clause versus a complete sentence. One needs to be vigilant, of course, for the effects of spelling on writing. Many students avoid words they cannot spell which, in effect, pulls their writing down to the level of their spelling. Others feel free to invent their spellings as needed but seem unaware that their spellings are nonstandard, which may be particularly true for those who spell phonetically. Because their spellings "look like they sound" they have difficulty identifying them as misspellings. Handwriting is interesting to observe in writing samples with the following questions in mind: Is the handwriting legible? Do the lines seem shaky or firm? Is there an unusual pencil grip? Does the writer steady the paper with the nonwriting hand or not seem to notice the need to do so? Is the paper slanted? Does the writer move his or her hand or the paper while moving along a line or keep the paper in place and rotate the writing hand at the wrist? Do letter formations suggest appreciation of distinctive features? For instance, does the writer seem to appreciate that the vertical part of an "h" in cursive or manuscript print must touch the curved portion to distinguish it from a small L followed by N? Is there a clear distinction between h and n in print showing appreciation of the distinguishing feature— the ascending line? Does the writer know how to connect the letters "b" and "r" to the next letter? A final question asks about automaticity of skills in writing. Is the writer spending time recalling letters and/or spellings that could be addressed to thinking and communicating ideas. What is automatic and what requires excessive thinking in the writing process for this adolescent? When peers have mastered the basic skills and gone on to develop their communication and style on paper, is the adolescent in question still working on all levels of language? More diagnostic questions to use when observing students' writing can be found in Box 6–3.

Educational Records Bureau Writing Assessment, level III (1997) for grades 10–12 gives a persuasive writing prompt and assesses topic development organization, support, sentence structure, word choice, mechanics, and total writing. Poteet (1998) reported a lack of psychometric data but the aspects of writing seem appropriate.

The *IDEA Reading and Writing Proficiency Test* (Amori, Dalton, & Tighe, 1993) for grades 3–12 can be used with the oral proficiency test for those with limited English proficiency.

The *CTB Writing Assessment* (1993) for grades 9–12.9 assesses personal expression, narrative, informative and persuasive writing resulting in national percentiles, NCEs and stanines.

The *Stanford Writing Assessment Program*, second edition (Harcourt Brace Educational Measurement of the Psychological Corporation, 1991) assesses description, narrative, exposition and persuasive writing.

BOX 6–3: *Diagnostic Questions About Writing*

1. How does the writer begin to write? Does the writer need to think first and plan? Or does the writer prefer to begin producing and then revise? Does this vary with the type of writing or topic?
2. Do they seem to generate ideas fluently or not?
3. How does the timed condition affect their writing?
4. Can the writer narrow an assigned topic? Do they?
5. Is there a main idea or event in their writing? Or just a list of ideas?
6. Is the writing organized?
7. Is there elaboration and complexity or just "bare bones?"
8. Does the writer change the style of writing when needed for different purposes?
9. Does the effort of handwriting and/or conscious spelling interfere in writing?
10. Is the writer avoiding needed or effective words because of spelling?

The *Writing Process Test* (Warden & Hutchinson, 1992) looks at development of the topic (purpose and focus; audience, vocabulary, style, tone, support and coherence) along with fluency (sentence structure, grammar, capitalization/punctuation and spelling. Kimmel (1998) suggested that this test would be a better tool for teaching than used for "high stakes decisions." He commented that this test would give students a good tool for self-evaluation of their writing.

Assessing Spelling

Moats (1994) describes spelling as a "multifaceted linguistic skill that integrates and depends on phonological, morphological, semantic, and orthographic knowledge;" making it clear that spelling difficulties "usually coexist with disorders of oral language," and that spelling can be a "visible record of language processing" (p.334, p.333). Assessing adolescents spelling (see Box 6–4) can provide insight into what they have noticed about language, particularly at the syllable and sound levels, and how that reflects what they do in pronouncing or in reading

---

BOX 6–4: *Diagnostic Questions for Spelling*

1. Do oral pronunciations show attention to syllables?
   (a) Are weak syllables neglected (computer, behind, invisible), pronounced?
   (b) Can the student rapidly repeat phonologically challenging words?
   (c) Can the student identify the number of syllables in a spoken word?
2. Does the student show awareness of sounds in words?
   (a) Can the student produce three rhyming words for a one syllable word?
   (b) Can the student identify a word when spoken with first sound segmented from the rhyming pattern (i.e., make the closure to find the word?)?
   (c) Can the student identify first sound and segment a word into first sound and remaining rhyming pattern?
   (d) Can the student segment a one syllable word into its constituent sounds?
   (e) Can the student build a word by adding sounds? (ar car cart)
3. What is the student's whole word memory like? For oral vocabulary? For spelling?
   (a) Can the student remember words but not break them into syllables or sounds?

(continued)

BOX 6–4: *(continued)*

    (b) Can the student read or spell a new word by analogy to a known word? ("Use this word 'cart' to figure out this word—part.")

  4. Does the student know the sounds of written consonants? Especially N, M, S?

  5. Can the student reverse the above processes and tell a letter for a sound?

  6. Can the student produce a new word by changing the first letter on request (in listening? in reading?)?

  7. Does the student show word confusions in spelling a correctly spelled but different word?

  8. What percentage of misspellings will elicit the correct word on a spell checker on a computer?

  9. What proportion of misspellings are phonetically correct?

10. What proportion of misspellings show structural errors (omissions, additions or reordering of letters and sounds?

11. Can the student identify his/her misspellings?

12. Can the student read the word the way it was misspelled?

13. Can the student spell a word by analogy to another word (i.e., use the shared pattern)?

14. What single consonants are misspelled? Consonant clusters? Consonant digraphs?

15. What long vowels are misspelled? Short vowels? Vowel digraphs?

16. Do misspellings reflect an attempt to recall the visual aspects of the word? Are there syllable omissions?

phonologically challenging words. Learning to spell *is* language learning and needs the same hospitality as the other language processes. Speech-language pathologists can and should contribute to the teaching and learning of spelling. They have been actively learning about phonologic awareness important in spelling (Lindamood, 1994), in identifying patterns in speech and oral language, and in directing children's attention to regular patterns in language. These are pertinent clinical skills that can be helpful in diagnosing and remediating language problems inherent in spelling.

When spellings are collected and analyzed, one may notice that many adolescents' misspellings are typical of young children and that there is a pattern of delay more than deviancy. Like their peers with stronger language learning skills, students with language learning problems will have difficulty learning to spell R controlled vowels, vowel digraphs, unstressed vowels (the schwa) and in doubling consonants. Students identified with dyslexia typically learn to spell in a phonetically correct fashion by second or third grade but have more difficulty with consonant blends, vowel–sonorant combinations, unstressed vowels and spellings that reflect complex relationships among morphology, phonology and orthography (Moats, 1994; Viise, 1992). It is most productive in assessing spelling to combine a formal test with a spelling analysis including misspellings from the test and from writing samples to uncover patterns.

The spelling subtest of the *Kaufman Test of Educational Achievement* (Kaufman & Kaufman, 1985) provides results in standard scores, grade level and percentiles based on grades 1–12. There is a format for error analysis (prefixes, suffixes, syllable patterns, vowel spellings and consonants) but there are only two to three examples for each pattern.

The *Test of Written Spelling*, fourth edition (TWS-R) (Larsen, Hammill, & Moats, 1999) provides two forms and is appropriate for students through grade 12. They have apparently eliminated the predictable–unpredictable spelling distinction that, in practice, was not helpful. *The Test of Written Language*, third edition, also results in spelling scores but, as in the TWS-R there is no attempt at analysis. The WRAT-III and achievement tests often include spelling lists with few examples of each pattern. There are also tests in which students are asked to select the correct spelling from an array that seems more like a sight word reading measure.

■□ SUMMARY

These reflections suggest that formal testing provides standardized measures that help us understand how adolescents compare with others at their age or grade level. The resulting scores can help us measure change and/or evaluate program plans or intervention methods. They can also inform adolescents about their strengths and weaknesses. Formal testing can also provide rich informal observations if one compares performances among various measures and notices how adolescents proceed in formal testing. These tests provide an opportunity to observe adolescents in various kinds of learning tasks. Formal testing can produce very limited information, however, if one simply records right and wrong answers along with final standardized scores. Farmer and Nesbit (2000) stated that "Assessment must not rely primarily on formal, standardized measures of performance at one point in time. Instead, assessment must be a process that integrates data from a variety of sources using a variety of methods" (p. 38). The combination of formal and informal assessment seems to yield a more useful measure of adolescents' abilities than does exclusive dependence on one or the other of these approaches to testing.

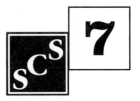

Principles and Issues in Intervention

Adolescents who struggle in school need guidelines for learning and direct instruction for applying those guidelines. Too often academic approaches identify those with natural abilities in school learning and screen out those who don't naturally know how to proceed in their studies. Just as natural athletes are identified and nurtured with many opportunities to play while those with less talent stay on the bench, the students who don't automatically create effective strategies on their own sometimes get left behind. A study strategies class for adolescents has offered one way to ensure that students learn specific ways to study under the structure of general guidelines. This class has evolved over a fifteen year period from first engaging a group of students in a variety of learning activities for daily sessions over one week to students' attending twice a week over a six week summer course that allows more time for active rehearsal of new strategies and flexibility in adjusting to students' needs from class to class. A study workbook was added to the in-class work to make strategies explicit and available for review during the school year. A parent meeting midway through the course also became necessary to involve and train parents to help students transfer these strategies to homework efforts.

This class is a compromise and study strategies are more effectively taught and reinforced when they are needed in each class. There is an advantage, however, in focusing on study strategies as an introduction to ways to study that can then be reactivated by teachers without their taking much time to teach them. Therefore, one way of helping students is a short study strategies course followed by guided use in school classes. The learning principles are presented as guiding principles for study in this course and, ideally, are woven throughout classes. There are many strategies taught, of course, but the principles can provide the underpinning for studying effectively.

■□ THE LEARNING PRINCIPLES

The learning principles presented in this chapter are "caught," taught and practiced throughout the course. It is important to engage students in activities that elicit natural understanding and use of these principles in their out-of-school lives—to "catch" them illustrating the principles thus creating a shared understanding and focus. The students' prior experience becomes a reference point for discussions of the principles.

Many of the adolescents who enroll in the course have been successful in athletics and provide illustrations of the "warming up" and "more than one way to skin a cat" principles. These youngsters regularly observe their opponents before a game, for instance, in order to plan or revise their strategies. Michael, a young man described in Chapter 4, applied good learning principles in football without being aware of the efficacy of applying, in school learning, these same natural ways of processing new information. The learning principles serve as a bridge between real world strategies and academic learning and have evolved from shoulder-to-shoulder, problem solving encounters with adolescents.

"Catching" the Principles

There are several ways to introduce students to the learning principles. They can be illustrated in cartoons (see Figures 7–1 through 7–10) posted in learning settings for easy reference during discussions or learning projects. It is effective for a speech-language pathologist or educator to "catch" a student illustrating good learning skills and point to the pictured version of the principle that has just been demonstrated. For instance, when a student suggests a different way to solve a math problem, provides a novel view of an event in history or poses an unusual question about an experiment in science, the "more than one way to skin a cat" principle can be identified ("That's a creative way to look at it, Adam. You are showing that there is often more than one way to 'skin a cat,' more than one way to do something or to look at something. That's helpful when you are learning."). It is important to mark these spontaneous illustrations of the learning principles to enhance awareness of and give a name to natural ways of proceeding that can also have validity in school learning.

Evoking Principles with Probes

Another way of introducing the principles includes using the following probes to evoke pertinent examples that can lead to an explanation of each principle.

1. Have you ever started through a buffet line, filled your plate with items and then come to your favorite food and wished you had looked over the whole array before making your choices? (Warm up)
2. How does your family store the various tools you have? (More than one way to skin a cat.)
3. If you worked the late shift at a restaurant, were busy until the end of the evening, what would you have to consider in closing up? (Wheat from chaff)
4. When parents discuss your using the family car, what is one point they might make?
   Why? (What–So what?)
5. Suppose they gave two demonstrations on the Food Channel: How to make a new kind of peanut butter sandwich and how to cook standing rib roast. Which demonstration would probably be easier to follow and why? (Old–New balance)
6. Suppose you came home one afternoon, as usual, and all the living room furniture was gone. What would you say? (Ask questions)
7. When you were getting ready to take the written driver's test, how did you make sure you had learned the information? (Test yourself)
8. I have some statistics about teenage driving and I would like you to teach this information to a partner. You have 5 minutes to do so. If your partner does well, you both will be given bonus points for your class grade. (After five minutes, ask the two students in each pair to write all that they recall from this lesson.) (Tutor–Tutee principle)
9. When parents talk to their children, they often seem to be "lecturing" about something that is causing a problem. Please recall a "lecture" you have heard from an adult or heard a friend telling about. Write what the lecture was about (one or two words only) and then explain the point the adult was trying to make. (Topic-Point)
10. Consider this. You are driving and have a flat tire. You have no spare tire and no cell phone. What would you do? (Problem solving)

The principles elicited with the probes and discussion are then made visible in posters and can be explained more thoroughly and reinforced as they are needed in lessons. For the less visual learner, the principles can be listed with a written explanation and examples given for each principle.

Identifying Principles in Regular Assignments

After having highlighted natural application of the principles, an instructor can observe students' illustrating principles during regular homework assignments and remind students of those principles as they work. The usual introduction of new lessons typically includes "warm-up" discussion to elicit background information and establish a context for specific information. Teachers could label this part of the lesson as the "warm-up" to help students appreciate this principle in use. Teachers could regularly include a discussion of pertinent principles when reviewing homework to see what "ways to skin a cat" were used, what problem solving strategies were necessary, and so forth. Identifying pertinent principles as a part of daily work encourages students to reflect on the learning process and particularly helps adolescents with language and learning difficulties. They could become aware of when and how to use the principles where they are needed most—in their regular school work. Learning principles are then integrated into school scripts.

Warm up for Learning

The athletes we have mentioned who intuitively know how to respond on the court or the field are often comfortable with the fast pace of sports and may be less naturally inclined to pause and reflect within a slower paced academic lesson. There are analogous principles in the two settings, however, that can create a shared perspective in communicating with our adolescent clients. The principle of "warming up" before active sports is well accepted, for instance. Young athletes appreciate the need to prepare their bodies and their minds for sport that provides the precedent for the "warm-up" exercises in listening, reading, writing and thinking for school (see Figure 7–1).

When students complain, in the learning interview, that teachers talk too fast or cover too much material in a lesson, they need to know that previewing the material beforehand would provide a good warm-up for listening. Adolescents who do not go into a game without looking over the field, sizing up their opponents, and mentally reviewing new plays, do not realize that a similar approach would help them in studying. Teachers typically elicit students' background information before lessons: writing the topic and asking for related words; creating a web with the topic and subtopics to provide a visual picture; asking students to make predictions based on a list of vocabulary words all ways to "warm-up." Westby and Costlow (1991) suggested that teach-

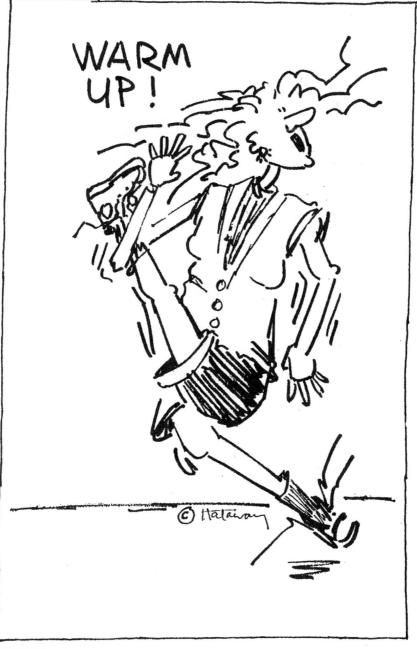

FIGURE 7-1

ers judge students' prior knowledge by their answers to questions in a warm-up period. She suggested that students' responses can show little knowledge about a pending topic (none to tangential knowledge), some knowledge (specific examples or defining characteristics of the concept) or much knowledge (show understanding of the concept within a superordinate category, provide a precise definition, give an analogous example, etc.). This diagnostic information can guide the teacher in communicating appropriately, but it can also provide needed background information and prepare students as they listen to others more familiar with the topic. Merritt, Barton, and Culatta (1998) suggested asking "life knowledge" questions (p.153) that would help create a "predicated topic," one that has relevance based on student's own information and examples elicited as background for discussion or reading. (Blank, Marquis, & Klimovitch, 1994; 1995; Blank & White, 1992).

The *PReP*, a prereading plan (Langer, 1981) presents a new concept or topic and asks students to first brainstorm ideas about that topic, then to add to initial thoughts, and finally, to reflect on ideas that have been discussed and are new for the students. This provides a warm-up along with monitoring of self-knowledge. Students need help in learning to warm up to academic tasks in these ways and in reminding that this is the way they proceed in sports and other out-of-school activities. They need to be aware of what teachers are doing and why in preparing them for lessons so they can begin to apply this principle independently in their learning. Although teachers have been "warming up" students for learning as a natural part of lessons, they have not always made this step explicit to students and they need to do so.

Gould (1991) suggested a variety of strategies that can serve as warm-ups to guide reading and writing. Construction of "probable passages" as predictions for a story are based on the earlier work of Wood (1984). In this approach, students are given an outline of story elements including the setting, characters, problem, solution and ending. They are also given key terms and phrases from the story to discuss and categorize under the appropriate story element. Using this information, they fill in blanks in a story frame provided by the teacher and construct a "probable" story. Then they read the actual story and compare it with their predicted story. Gould suggested that after guided practice with teacher-provided materials, students could be asked to scan stories and construct probable stories within small groups. Adolescents in this effort to practice the "warming up" principle, might enjoy concocting various possible scenarios and then comparing their predictions with the actual text. Teachers of young children often do something less stringent but with the same purpose by simply showing pictures in a story and eliciting guesses from children about the story. In both cases, the students are guided to "warm up" to facilitate comprehension in the reading of the story.

Other warm-up or prereading strategies described by Gould (1991) include 1) using semantic maps to guide students attention to specific parts of a story, naming characters (with spokes for listing different traits of each character), setting (with spaces for students to note locations and time) and so forth; 2) macro-cloze exercises in which students are given a story with a component missing and create their own setting, beginning, problem, reaction, and so forth. Various groups can create different parts and then assemble the parts to create a novel passage, which presumably can be contrasted with the reading of the original passage (Whaley, 1981); 3) various types of graphic organizers; and 4) text frames with details to be filled in by students. In all these instances the prereading activities evoke predictions to prepare students for reading.

The Directed Reading-Thinking Activity (Stauffer & Cramer, 1968; Stauffer, 1969) has long been used to encourage active reading and includes warming up by reading the title of a story followed by students' predicting what will happen in the story. They continue throughout a piece reading a paragraph at a time, predicting-reading-and-confirming or changing their predictions in light of new information. This active processing provides conscious practice in "warming up" with each prediction, which guides attention. Having a prediction in mind makes the reading easier if the text fits their assumptions or it causes readers to notice when the text does not fit. When these activities occur in a group, at risk students who may lack information about the topic can listen to others who are more informed and warm up for the topic so they can make some prediction. They can also notice when and how others revise predictions when confronted with new or conflicting information. The student whose devotion to first predictions, called "premature cognitive commitment" (Langer, 1989), may come to appreciate that new information often requires that one rethink and make a new prediction.

The *Request Procedure* (Manzo, 1969) has been suggested for those who "get 'lost' early" in the reading of a new selection (Blachowisc, 1994) p. 308. In this procedure the instructor and student take turns reading silently followed by asking questions of the other person. If the instructor's first questions are intended to establish the topic, this warm-up will facilitate comprehension.

The *K-W-L strategy* (Ogle, 1986; Carr & Ogle, 1987) asks students to brainstorm ideas then write what they already know or think about a topic under a column labeled *"know,"* then to list questions they have about that topic under a column labeled *"want* to find out" as two ways to warm up for their reading. After gathering information through reading, they report their findings under a *"learned"* column. This provides a structured warm-up for reading and writing.

The *SQ3R* (Robinson, F., 1962; Robinson, H., 1978) study strategy has as its first letter, S, which stands for surveying the chapter (followed by question, read, recite and review). Variations on this approach all stress the importance of "warming up" by surveying or previewing before reading. Even at risk adolescents typically look over the cover picture and note the title when selecting videos to rent. Naming such activities as "warm-ups," having the poster available as a visible reminder of this principle when it is needed, and practicing regular prereading or prelistening strategies can help youngsters consciously add this "warm-up" step to their school routines.

In his *"Muscle Reading"* approach, Ellis (1991) provides a mnemonic for the warm-up phase: "Pry Out Questions" which reminds the student to preview the entire reading assignment or engage in "Textbook Reconnaissance" (page vi), followed by outlining, and creating questions. This phase, in Ellis' strategy, is followed by "Rooting Up Answers " (read, underline, answer), and "Recite, Review and Review again." Ellis explains the need for this kind of active processing by stating that although texts have value, "Sometimes that value is so buried that extracting it requires skill and energy," and "muscle" in your reading approach (p. 98).

One middle school teacher regularly includes a test question that asks the title of the current chapter, to emphasize that her students should know what the chapter is about as a context for learning specific facts. Once warming up enters the shared vocabulary of students and educators, they can recognize many such opportunities to evoke this principle in learning (see Box 7–1).

BOX 7–1: *Ways To "Warm Up"*

1. Write the topic and elicit related words.
2. Create a web with topic and subtopics.
3. Provide vocabulary and ask for predictions.
4. Ask related "life knowledge" questions.
5. Use PReP for prereading.
6. Construct "probable passages."
7. Provide cloze passages for prediction
8. Vary kinds of graphic organizers and text frames.
9. Use DRTA to promote prediction.
10. Use the Request Procedure with first questions to show topic.
11. Use K-W-L to elicit prior knowledge and questions.
12. Promote surveying using SQ3R.
13. "Pry out questions" for "Muscle Reading."
14. Require students to know the title of the chapter.
15. Note "Warming Up" and label it in regular school activities.

There's More Than One Way to Skin a Cat

During discussions or brainstorming, a student might suggest a new way of doing something or looking at an issue that presents the opportunity to introduce the poster bearing the adage "There is more than one way to skin a cat" (see Figure 7–2). Using the students' varied

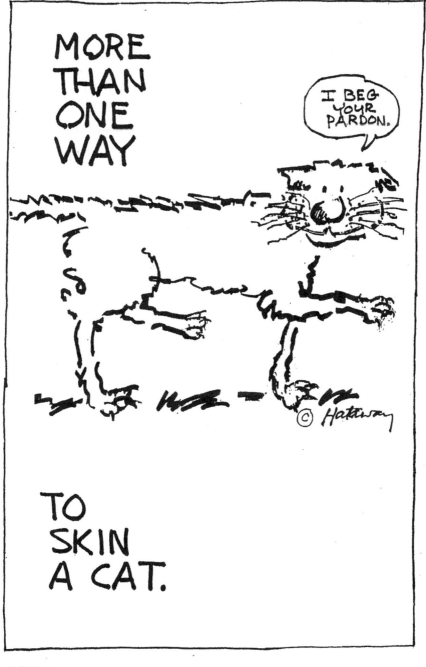

FIGURE 7-2

comments as examples of flexible thinking, the instructor or adult collaborator can show the value of various approaches to learning. Adolescents with language and learning difficulty often approach an academic challenge as though there is only one answer or solution— one they probably do not know. They waste time, then, trying to find or remember that one perfect answer when they could be exploring logical possibilities. Although they may show divergent thinking in other tasks, less successful students often do not apply it to school learning. Educators need to identify and celebrate the ability to think of various ideas for nonacademic problems to bring this principle to a conscious level. Generating possible fundraising projects for student trips; collecting reasons why students should be able to go off campus for lunch; discussing pros and cons of raising the driving age and similar topics might elicit varied examples of flexible thinking to illustrate the "More than one way to skin a cat" principle. This principle can be applied and named in mini-lessons within a process writing approach that teach various strategies for finding topics, for getting started in writing assignments, and/or for expanding language in writing. Students can be asked to quickly write three topics or three first sentences and then explain how they thought of ideas under this kind of pressure. Students having difficulty can learn from others and add strategies to their own repertoire for writing.

> "Well, I just thought about what Lori said in her story and that reminded me of the time we saw an accident on a ferris wheel. Last week, I couldn't think of a topic and I started look around the room. I saw a picture of a boat and that made me think of water. I started thinking of times when I was at the ocean but nothing came of that. Then I remembered seeing a movie about whales and how they travel so far with their babies. I decided to write a sad story about a baby whale getting lost along the way."

Adolescents who assume that more successful students produce ideas and answers without effort will learn from these discussions that other students are also stymied at times and must work at thinking of ways to solve learning problems. It is helpful to hear other students explain their learning and hear their "thinking language" (Nelson, 1998, p. 7) especially for those students who have limited awareness of their own thinking. At risk youngsters can add to their own ways of "skinning a cat" by listening to others.

Besides brainstorming at the beginning of or discussing strategies after a writing project, introducing the concept of "good mistake" is helpful for impressing the "more than one way ... " principle during learning. Knowing that one can make a mistake that shows good thinking is a new idea for many students who think only in terms of right or wrong answers. Adult collaborators regularly rewarding good logic even when an answer is wrong encourages expression of multiple views in learning. To truly appreciate that there is "more than one way to skin a cat" students need to know that an idea that may not work can lead to a better idea or contribute to a problem solving process by eliminating one idea that need not be considered again. Kriegel and Patler (1991) quoted a company president who advised his people to make "at least two mistakes a week" (p. 196) to show that they were trying new things. Apparently this successful business executive felt that one must stumble through some less than great ideas to find the better "ways to skin a cat." Adolescents need to know and value this principle.

Lewis and Greene (1982) explain that those who are "Helicopter Pilots" will be comfortable in brainstorming and using a somewhat intuitive approach to problem solving and adolescents comfortable with this natural approach may simply need to know where this can be helpful in school. The "Pathfinders" who prefer a systematic way of working through a task may need to stretch their natural style to include more ways "to skin a cat." Adolescents with either style need experience with convergent problems that lend themselves to the more disciplined, methodical approach favored by Pathfinders and practice in proceeding in this way. They also need many divergent tasks that provide practice in generating many ideas before limiting oneself to a solution. In this principle, as with all the others, the style of the students needs to be considered. Some will naturally demonstrate some principles more than others and need to be led to learn new ways of proceeding (see Box 7–2).

We make the point that a learner should try a variety of ways to solve school problems, but easily frustrated adolescents or those who have had limited prior success may have difficulty applying the principle on their own. When encountering stumbling blocks in an assignment, these students will need direct help in developing and using a list of strategies before they may be expected to generate ideas on their own. We can't leave adolescents with just a principle and assume they can apply it.

A high school teacher expressed concern that her students with learning disabilities waited for her help in a guided study hall period without first trying anything on their own. She worried that she was

---

BOX 7–2: *Ways to "Skin a Cat"*

1. Note and list varied ideas in brainstorming or discussion of homework.
2. Brainstorm and discuss ideas for writing topics, for getting started, for expanding basic thoughts, and so forth.
3. Value "good " mistakes that show good thinking.
4. Provide both convergent and divergent tasks.
5. Teach various strategies through mini-lessons and then require that students use more than one.

simply "dragging them through their daily assignments" and they were not really learning. She felt overwhelmed as she tried to attend to each student's needs and somewhat "used" because the students seemed to expect her to do all the work. This teacher and I collaborated to design a better process for helping students within this study hall period.

The teacher listed typical assignments students brought to the study hall along with the common difficulties presented by these assignments. Students were frequently asked, for instance, to read and answer questions at the end of a chapter and they often had difficulty finding the answers. Having identified this particular problem, the teacher taught a mini-lesson on ways to find answers, including determining a key word in the question and finding that word in the book's index to quickly locate the page where the answer might be found. She also taught students how to turn the question into a fact statement to highlight the main idea of the question and to serve as the beginning of their answer ("Read the question, then, 'Gentlemen, start your answers' "). For the question: "Why did Jefferson think the Louisiana Purchase was beneficial to the new nation?" the students learned to restate the question: "Jefferson thought the Louisiana Purchase would be beneficial to the new nation in these ways ... " This directed the students to the facts they were looking for in the text. This teacher went on to identify other problems and teach strategies through mini-lessons. After each mini-lesson the strategies were summarized and listed on charts around the room. Students then practiced using the strategies under the guidance of the teacher as the final step in the mini-lesson. New strategies were added to the chart as they came up in discussion or in subsequent lessons. The first plan to facilitate independence in their schoolwork in this guided study hall, then, was for students to have charts available that labeled specific homework problems and displayed strategies taught for them to use in solving those problems. After the mini-lesson, display of the chart and practicing the strategies, the teacher created study sheets or "contracts" to guide the students in their work during the guided study period. These study sheets required that students write their assignment (chapter, page, task), explain in writing the specific problem they were having with that assignment, and write what solutions from the wall charts they had already tried. They were required to show that they had consulted the lists of strategies posted in their study hall and had attempted to use at least one of theses strategies before calling on the teacher for help.

In the spirit of the problem solving process, the teacher tried this contract plan with the students and found that the study sheets were impractical. They required too much time and writing, so she created specialized study sheets for typical assignments (see Box 7–3). The strategies for problems identified in those kinds of lessons and taught in mini-lessons were listed right on the sheet. Students were still required to describe their assignment and their particular problem as in the original design, but now they simply had to check which strategy they had tried on their own. If their problem was not solved by applying one of the strategies previously taught and listed on their study sheet, the teacher would consult with them. After the use of these specialized study sheets became routine, the teacher began to require that students try *more than one solution* before she became involved. This was a very direct way to encourage the application of multiple strategies. The students had to show daily that "There is more than one way to skin a cat" and to apply this principle in their school work. This process also demonstrated to students that they had a responsibility to do something before consulting the teacher for help; that this was a shoulder-to-shoulder effort. It seemed important in this project for students to understand that explaining what they had tried would be effective in school problem solving and in so doing they were actually practicing a good procedure for being an employee—that when they first try solutions on their own before consulting their boss with a problem, they are saving time and proving that they are valuable employees. Practical students do not always see the relationship between school and work and pointing this out to them may make school efforts more meaningful.

BOX 7–3: *Study Sheet for Finding Answers to Questions*

Name_____ Date_____
My assignment is for _____(name the class),
Chapter ____Page___
I have to do the following _____
_____
_____

On my own I have tried the following strategies for finding answers:

_____ **1.** I turned the question into a statement. This statement can help me form my answer.
_____ **2.** I underlined key words in the question and looked those words up in the index to find the page I need.
_____ **3.** I decided the topic of the question and looked for a subtitle in the chapter that was about that topic. I looked in that section for the answer.

I have tried the above strategies but still have a problem. This is my problem:
_____
_____

I need to consult with the teacher.

Separate Wheat from Chaff

The third principle (Figure 7–3) directs students to separate "Wheat from Chaff" in the information they hear, see, read and write. Students are introduced to the concept of winnowing wheat with descriptions of primitive people tossing baskets of wheat into the air to separate the valuable wheat that falls into the basket to be saved, from the less valuable chaff that blows away in the wind or falls through the holes in the basket. The instructor needs to stress the reason for this winnowing process—to separate the important from the unimportant and relate this to listening and reading for school.

Adolescents are often impatient with overly verbose friends or parents and comments such as "Cut to the chase, will you?" or "Please, Mom, get to the point!" will probably sound familiar to them. This can serve as an example of the "chaff" which they don't want to hear and their preference for unembroidered "wheat." These quotes might help adolescents bridge from winnowing wheat to their own daily processing

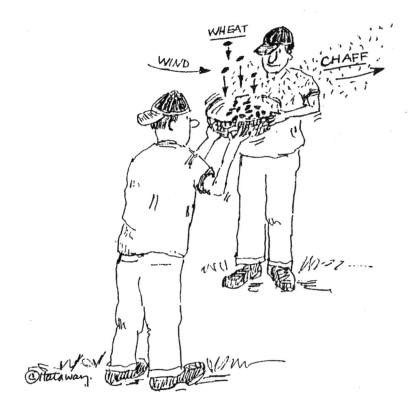

FIGURE 7-3

of information. Real world scenarios can be described and discussed for their most important features, their "wheat," so that students can recognize their natural tendency to focus on the critical elements in what they see or hear. (What do you notice first when you go to a party? What do you want to know? What are the important last minute instructions given by the coach in a huddle? What is critical in training for a long bicycle ride?)

A group of young adolescents was discussing what they notice and how these observations guide their understanding in social situations. The question, "How can you tell when your mother is angry?" caused one student to say, "Well, she walks out of the room." In this case, the walking did not seem to clearly represent "wheat," so I said, " I assume that she also walks out of the room when she is not angry. How can you tell when she is walking out of a room angry?" This young man paused and then said, "Well, when she's mad, she walks real hard." The discussion then focused on all the things the mother did during that short walk that were not pertinent and could be considered "chaff" as opposed to the "hard walking" that was definitely "wheat" in this situation and needed to be noticed. This presented a example of the young man's natural understanding of "wheat versus chaff" in observing his mother.

Showing Wheat in the Request Procedure

The *Request Procedure* (Manzo, 1969) has been discussed for its "warming-up" qualities but it also provides opportunities for identifying "wheat" in reading. As an instructor and student read silently together and take turns creating questions, the instructor selects the important information to question first, rather than to ask about minor details. The instructor can also illustrate the relative importance of information by storing and recalling "wheat" while having to check back in the text for the "chaff."

Listening for Wheat

There is an exercise, "Listening for the wheat," that asks students to listen or read and write all the facts they recall. (See discussion of Lisa in Chapter 4). After they exhaust their memory for facts, students select the three facts they consider the most important or "wheatiest" facts and explain their choices. Hearing the reasons others give for deciding on the most important facts allows less successful students to appreciate others' processing of meaning. Students with pragmatic language problems in particular can profit from this discussion as others explain their clues for noting "Wheat" including words, gestures, facial expressions and other signals in conversations or in reading.

Noticing Signals for Wheat

A teacher or SLP can invite students to listen and watch a mini-lecture to find signals for "wheat" in the speaker's delivery: using a louder voice ... repeating a fact or name ... pausing for effect ... numbering facts ... identifying causes and effects ... and so forth. Students can do a mini-research project to discover how different teachers signal important information. A favorite professor of mine, for example, always first reviewed information from a prior lecture and then signaled new and important information by saying "Having said that ... " and the students started taking notes at that point. This phrase served as a "snap back" signal to those who recognized the review as old information and began to drift. Those who have normal vision but use recorded texts designed for the visually impaired need to practice listening for a "snap back" signal when there are lengthy descriptions of illustrations that they do not need. When they hear the phrase, "Return to text" they should return to an active listening and notetaking mode for the "wheat" that will follow.

Students and teachers can identify wheat versus chaff after observing or participating in science experiments to show their understanding that all observations are not equally important. Developing notetaking skill is, of course, highly dependent on this wheat-chaff principle; therefore, helping students learn the concept of "wheat" and to recognize specific signals in both oral and written language seems critical. Those with language learning difficulties may need many examples in order to understand and apply the "wheat versus chaff" principle in their own listening and reading.

Noting Key Words

There is an exercise, *Noting Key Words* (See Box 7–4), in which the instructor selects a list of ten sentences, perhaps main ideas that can introduce or be used for reviewing a lesson, and determines the key words needed to represent and recall the basic meaning of each sentence.

The instructor reads each sentence aloud and tells the students they may write a specified maximum number of key words (numbers in the parentheses in Box 7–4), to guide their recall of the sentence. Limiting the number of words should cause a conscious choice of important words. The sentences can be repeated several times to allow the students to focus on the relative importance of words rather than to stress their memory for the sentences. After all sentences have been read, and key word notes written, the students are asked to recall and write the original sentence using their key words to guide them. Students are then shown the original sentence to check their recall of sentences based on their choice of key words. They discuss which key words were chosen, why they were chosen and how well these words helped them recall the information. This is a good demonstration of how determining "wheat from chaff" guides thinking in notetaking.

BOX 7–4: *Noting Key Words*

Ellen Foster was the *brave heroine* of Kate *Gibbons's first novel*. (7)
The *main character* in the *first novel* has been *likened* to *Holden Caulfield*. (7)

Blinking Jack Stokes was *forty*, *twice* the age of his *bride*. (6)

Gibbons's second novel, a *Virtuous Woman*, presents a *multilayered picture* of two *ill-matched people* who somehow *created* a *marriage*. (11)

The *Sue Kaufman Prize* for *First Fiction* was given to Kate *Gibbons* for her *Ellen Foster* and she also *received accolades* from *Walker Percy* and *Audrey Wetly*, two outstanding and well-known *writers*. (15)

A variation of this exercise, *Key Word Delay*, asks students to take key word notes with the same constraint to write only a given number of words for each sentence, but they are asked to recall the sentence after a delay, perhaps after several days or a week. Students discover that, after a long period, they might reconstruct a different sentence and change the meaning of the original sentence. This exercise shows students the importance of reviewing notes soon after class each day by turning them into sentences that reflect the original meaning. College students with learning problems are advised to plan a regular slot in their study schedules to allow for this daily reconstructing of notes after each class, while the information is fresh and they can use their key word notes to accurately recall the points made in class.

Writing with "Wheat" and "Chaff" in Mind

After brainstorming or free writing students have to make decisions about what they want to include or discard in their writing. They have to focus on their purpose and main idea to determine what is wheat. Donald Graves (1983) suggested that after gathering information for a writing piece, the writer should consider what question he or she is trying to answer. This certainly helps a writer develop a focus. Harvey (Harvey & Goudis, 2000) suggested the guiding question for writers, "What information will best help my reader understand the topic?" (p. 127)

Students often read aloud to check the clarity of their writing at many stages in the process, and presumably ask themselves, "Did I make my point? Was it clear?" or "Is the 'wheat' coming through? Is there chaff that needs to be eliminated?" In writing conferences, students often learn from the questions of conference partners when important information has been omitted or is not clear. When students outline their papers, write summaries, and throughout most of the writing process, the wheat-chaff issue is clearly a guiding principle.

Because effective learning requires attention to the main idea, critical features, primary causes, important outcomes, and so on, students clearly need to appreciate the "wheat versus chaff" concept. They need to be made aware of signals that guide them to "wheat" and be directed within specific learning tasks to apply this principle. As with all the principles, it is helpful to have a name, "wheat versus chaff" to highlight awareness and to guide discussion of active learning (see Box 7–5).

BOX 7–5: *Ways to Separate Wheat from Chaff*

1. Discussing real life situations: parties, coaches' instructions, identifying parents' moods, and so forth.
2. The Request Procedure: showing "wheat" through questions and answers.
3. Listening for wheat: recalling and prioritizing facts.
4. Observing teacher's signals.
5. Discussing observations in science experiments.
6. Noting key words: Limiting selection of words for notetaking.
7. Key word delay: Limiting selection and recall after delay.
8. Consider "wheat-chaff" issues throughout the writing process.

Ask "What" and "So What?"

Once, during a mini-lecture about study strategies, I paused at an appropriate stopping point and asked the group, "Now what point have I been making here? What have I been trying to tell you about studying?" The students seemed hesitant to risk being wrong but, after I reassured them by saying, "Just say what it sounded like to you. I saw you and know you were listening. What point do you think I am making ... tell any little part you remember." A few brave students volunteered to answer and they were basically correct. They seemed clear on the concept that had been explained and they seemed to appreciate their obligation to know *what* had been said. I then asked them to explain the new concept in light of the general topic and other comments, that is, the reason to make this point:

> Okay that's good. That is the point I was making. Now, 'So what?' What does this point have to do with the topic? And what does it have to do with the other points I have made today? You remembered the point and that's good, but now tell me why I made this point?

This question was greeted with complete silence. The students seemed not to hesitate, in this instance, because they feared being wrong. Rather, they seemed genuinely surprised by the question. A "So what?" discussion seemed foreign to this particular group of adolescents perhaps because they seemed to focus their responsibility on collecting, remembering and reporting facts on demand—on the "What" part of teacher's lectures and their reading without asking the "So what" question.

The need for stressing the "What–So what" principle (see Figure 7–4) was evident on another occasion when a ninth grader had answered questions for a science assignment and was quite proud at having finished his assignment on time, which was a notable accomplishment as he was generally disorganized about schoolwork. His celebration should have been tempered, however, because he clearly had a very superficial view of the task. A review of his homework showed that he had simply copied a sentence that shared a key word with each question. He was asked to explain what he thought he was supposed to do in that science assignment. ("What do you think your teacher wanted you to do? What was your job in that assignment?") He answered quickly, "To find the answers and memorize them." It was clear that this young man meant to find a "What" in the book without any appreciation for the "So what?"

Attending to Sentence Level

Attention to individual facts is often seen when students are asked to summarize a passage from an expository text. They seemed to recall each idea without showing understanding of the theme or main idea that tied those sentences together. The adolescents in the study strategies class and the young man with the limited view of science homework were identified because of known learning difficulties and were typical of many at risk youngsters in their apparent focus on sentence level processing without appreciation of the overall meaning or purpose of the passage or task. They seemed stuck at the level of sentences rather than progressing to efficient processing of paragraphs or longer discourse. Unfortunately, these students are asked to manage language beyond the sentence level in middle school, high school and college. They need help in appreciating the "What–So what" connections in order to do so.

Attending to "So What" in the Real World

Many of these same adolescents seem to regularly ask the "So what?" in their casual interchanges. When they enter a conversation late and hear a provocative comment, they would naturally ask, "What happened? Why is he so mad?" suggesting that they realize they need a context of the statement. They know, in this case, what was said and they naturally ask themselves and others "So what?" to understand

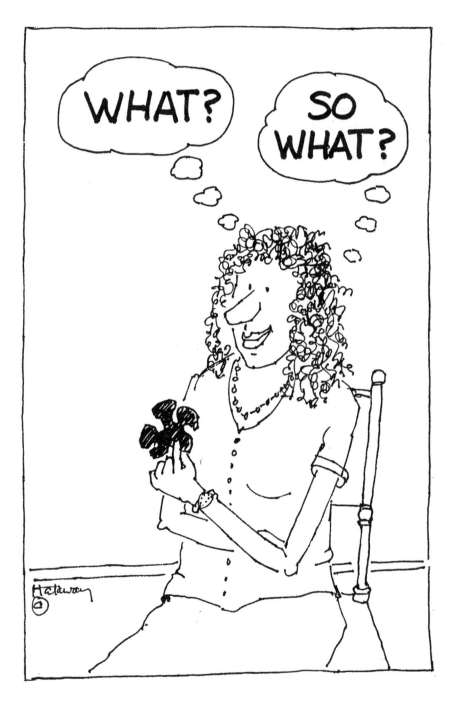

FIGURE 7-4

why this comment was made. Harvey and Goudis (2000) described a teacher's capitalizing on the natural question of middle school students at the beginning of an account of the Titanic's sinking. They immediately wondered "why" this ship sank. This is a good example of knowing the fact (it sank) and asking "So what?" to go beyond memorizing to understanding. The teacher guided the students to circle words in their text that helped explain this tragedy. They put comments or further questions in the margins. These same authors encouraged readers to place stick-on notes on the pages to show connections between what they read and an experience it reminded them of or a fact they knew from their world knowledge. This seems a very concrete way to encourage students to learn and remember facts in relation to other things they know—to make sense of what they are reading and learning.

Highlighting Connections

Teachers need to highlight connections among and between statements and to the overall topic to help students go beyond sentence level processing and there are a variety of ways to do this. Merritt and Culatta (1998) suggested that teachers "facilitate connections among ideas or sentences" by highlighting connecting elements while they are "telling, explaining and discussing a narrative." (p. 300). Reading text aloud with pauses for making cohesive ties (" ... the other one? To whom are they referring?") and allowing students to respond with referents is very effective in directing attention to the connections among ideas in narratives and expository text and can take students beyond the processing of isolated sentences to making connections between and among thoughts. Good readers naturally make these connections but teachers need to make the connections explicit for those without this talent. They need to be taught what others, often teachers, do without thinking.

I have described elsewhere a strategy for helping students attend to cohesion in text. This activity starts with a "just me" phase in which I, as the instructor, take responsibility for modeling the process of noting cohesive ties. I read aloud as the students follow along. When I encounter a word that requires that the reader tie that word to a referent ("The governor proposed the idea of building a bridge. *This idea* was quite popular."), I pause and ask a question that highlights the implied word or phrase that needs to be connected to the referent ("*This* idea? What idea?"). Then I think aloud while finding the referent ("Oh, they're referring to *the idea that the governor proposed about building a bridge*. That's the idea they are referring to."). After modeling this process of noticing words that imply a referent and then identifying the referent, the process moves to a collaborative stage, "me then you," in which I, as instructor, simply identify the word or phrase where a tie must be made. I read that word with a questioning tone ("*This idea*? What idea? What do they mean?), and the students are to find and explain the referent, thus making the tie. There may be a need for an advanced "me then you again" step here, in which I tell the students whether there is a tie, but do not identify the exact words. The students must find the words that imply a tie and make the tie to the referent. Finally, in the effort to direct students' attention to cohesion in texts, the "just you" stage is reached. In this stage, the students decide if there are cohesive ties to be made in the text or not and, if so, where they occur in terms of the exact words that imply a tie to the referent, and then the student explains what the words refer to (Tattershall, 1994b, p. 69). It is always effective in language learning lessons such as these, of course, to use students' writing to identify cohesive ties and referents. This "catching" of ties in their own writing shows that this is a natural language process that they already know, except for the name. Naming the process makes it explicit.

Merritt, Barton and Culatta (1998) described lessons in which teachers helped students make connections among individual facts or comments by regularly reiterating the focus of the lesson that had been established in the introduction and by "asking students to articulate their own understanding of instructional goals" at the end of each discussion (p. 159). Without this help in connecting comments to topic, many students might otherwise focus on isolated comments for their own sake or go off on tangents without reference to the topic. The "What-So what?" principle seems to be at work in this effort to ensure that students know what is being said and how it relates to the topic at hand. These same meaning connections need to be demonstrated through discussions of stories, textbook topics, current events, and movies to remind students to think of new information in the context of overall meaning relationships. Other ways of demonstrating the "What-So what?" principle can be found in Box 7–6

BOX 7–6: *Ways To Show "What–So What?"*

1. Periodically stop in discussions and ask students to state the point being made and why.
2. Ask students to provide proof or clues from reading for answers.
3. Stop in discussions and tie individual points to each other and topic.
4. Model, highlight and guide students in identifying cohesive ties.
5. Engage students in responding to passages without clear referents.
6. Ask students to identify connections from text to real world experiences and knowledge or to other reading.

There is an interesting way to direct students to the importance of knowing the topic as a way of tying isolated facts together. One can present, on an overhead projector or in handouts, passages in which the topic and referents have not been established resulting in isolated facts that are unclear (see Box 7–7). We have presented them to students without comment and then asked for a retelling or even a drawing to illustrate the passage. The subsequent discussion can reveal a misconception without awareness. The student can draw a picture or offer an explanation without seeming to appreciate that they do not have enough information to make this conclusion. More aware students pause to show that they are confused and realize that the passages do not make sense.

It is effective to then add a topic sentence and to write pronoun references above the pronouns ("I forgot to make this clear. This is the topic and I will introduce people and concepts so that the sentences will make sense."). In the second passage below, students often can construct meaning from the words, "swarming, sprayed and sting" that evoke the topic of bees or wasps which can guide discussion of connecting the individual words or facts ("What") to topics in order to make sense and comprehend ("So what").

BOX 7–7: *No Topic–No Referents Exercise*

Passage One:

He was frantic. "She'll kill me!" he screamed. "I've got to find it or I'm in big trouble ... " She came out to see what all the noise was about. He said, "She's really going to kill me if I don't find it." She said, "Oh, she'll understand. Just tell her the truth." Then she went back inside the house. She said, "She has no idea what she's like. You're dead meat."

Passage Two:

She wanted to finish it but she couldn't see so she raised the shade to let in some light. Suddenly there were a million of them! She tried to knock it down but she missed, and they came swarming at her! She called for help and he came running from the kitchen. He went to get the spray and they sprayed and sprayed. Luckily, they did not sting them but what a scary experience. She didn't know that raising the blind was such a dangerous thing to do.

Appreciate the Old–New Balance

Bloom, Hood, and Lightbown (1974) studied the language of echolalic children, those who seemed to simply reproduce what others said rather than generating their own novel comments. These children rarely echoed the language that they knew well and could produce on their own or that which was too hard for them. They seemed most likely to repeat those phrases that contained elements that were known to them and in their repertoire of language forms but also included new language elements. It was as if the children needed old information that made the task of repeating seem possible, along with new elements that caught their ear, interested them and required extra processing. This old–new balance (see Figure 7–5) seems to describe the way most of us pay attention in many situations and to be pertinent to school learning. Students need a modicum of old information to feel comfortable and confident ("Yes, I recognize something here. I can handle this.") and to serve as a context for new learning. If the teacher starts a discussion by reviewing what has been said and/or invoking real world experience, this helps listeners get ready to process new information. Using this old–new balance model for best attention, the teacher must lay the groundwork with the old but must include something novel or new to provide a reason to listen. If the information is very familiar students will not listen very long. The same is true when there is an overload of new information. Students can only absorb so much new information, and, when they determine that there is too much new information to reasonably learn, they stop attending.

Maintaining Attention

Adolescents often report that they are bored in certain classes. This can sometimes mean that they already know about the topic and need the teacher to move more quickly to something new. However, with at risk adolescents, one has to explore this "bored" condition and what it means. Sometimes there is actually too much new information and they can't learn. When they are bombarded with new information it may feel as though the class is being taught in a foreign language and, because they can't follow the discussion, they become bored.

A child who was hearing impaired presented with a vocabulary knowledge and related background information that was so impoverished that his social studies text was impossible for him to understand. The author of his textbook presumed a certain background knowledge, and this boy did not have it. The teacher also presumed a base of information and, for this youngster, seemed to always start in the middle of a discussion, so he was lost. To restore an appropriate balance of old and new information, he required extensive help in acquiring needed old information as a context for the new concepts.

Understanding the Old-New Balance

Students and teachers need to understand the old–new balance and its significance in classroom learning. Teachers are presented with remarkable diversity in the information that students bring to lessons and they

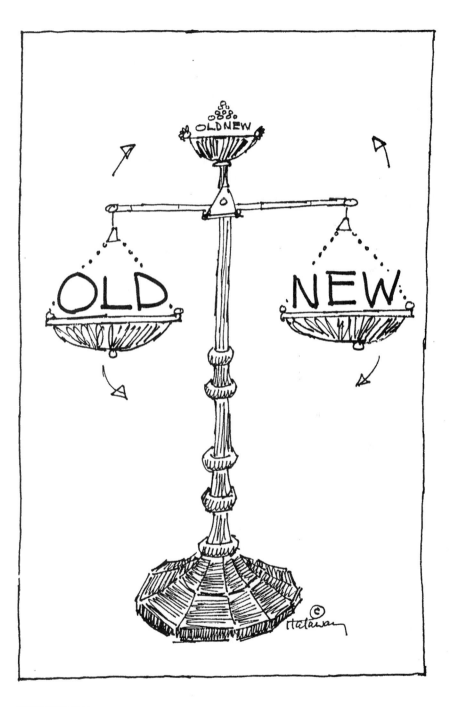

FIGURE 7-5

usually try to address the problem. When engaged in whole group instruction they identify those who conceptualize quickly because they have prior knowledge. To keep them alert for new information, they say to these students, "Now, stay with me, there is going to be more information coming." To those who are confused and perhaps overloaded with new information, they say, "Now, stay with me. I promise, this will make sense to you." Creative teachers sometimes manage to satisfy both groups, but it is hard. Many students need extra "priming" for lessons to give them the base of old information necessary for learning the new. If they are prepared in this way, they can attend to classroom discussion and learn. Of course, teachers regularly introduce new lessons in some way to allow students to activate what they already know about the subject in order to better understand. Comments from others with pertinent background information help provide background for those who do not have that old information, but the usual "warm-up" to new lessons is insufficient for students with significant gaps in their knowledge base.

Discussions of attention style regarding the balance of information can be provoked by observations during lessons. When explaining something to a student, and it is clear that they are tired of the old and want to move on, it is good for the instructor to acknowledge the student's body language that signals this attention style.

> I see that your eyes are beginning to wander around, you are nodding quickly, and shifting in your chair so I guess you want to move on? This is a good time for you to interrupt politely and paraphrase what I am saying to let me know that you understand. You might wait for a pause, a stopping place, and say, for example "So, you are saying that a phobia is a kind of unnatural fear?" That's a good way to get me to move on from old to new information. It also helps those who would like to be more sure before we move on. When they hear you explain the concept they will be comfortable about it.

Those students with the opposite attention style, a need for extensive old information and a thorough warm-up, need to know this about themselves. They may be the sequential learners who feel that they need to understand something thoroughly before going on to something else (see Lisa in Chapter 4). Or they may just be very careful people who like to feel securely grounded in a topic in order to listen. Students with this style need to know that a teacher may have a different, more fast-paced style than they prefer or there may be so much information to cover that it is necessary to go quickly.

Presenting Appropriate Balance

London (1993) seems to address the old–new balance in describing "appropriately challenging" nonroutine math problems for adolescents. A problem for which the student can quickly determine a solution is too easy in his approach. On the other hand, a problem for which the student has no idea how to even start and finds frustrating is inappropriately difficult. London suggests a scenario in which the balance is achieved: "The student reads the problem, has no clear idea what the solution is but has a few ideas about how to start, tries something and becomes clearer about the solution, eventually finds a good solution, and, from the processing of the problem realizes some ways he or she could have improved the process or solution." (p. 34)

Preferring Old or New Information

In addition to the need to balance old and new information as London described, there are personal styles to consider. Some students do not like extensive old information and seem to need novelty in order to sustain their best attention. They like a fast pace and are quickly bored when teachers review. A student with this attention style recognizes familiar information and quickly stops listening assuming that the information will be redundant. If this student knows about and can listen for a "snap back" signal, such as the "having said that" of a professor mentioned earlier, and begins listening again for new information this style may not present problems; however, few students know to learn these signals. They assume too quickly that the review is going to be boring, don't realize that they may need a review even if the information is familiar, and don't appreciate the review may provide a base for understanding new information.

One excellent math student reported that he often understood new problems as they were being shown on the board and would stop listening to the teacher's explanations. He admitted, however, that when he began doing the homework, he often realized that he had forgotten how to do the problems. This student was asked if he was irritated with those who needed extra explanation and asked many questions while the teacher was explaining the new problems. He agreed that he often wondered why they couldn't conceptualize math as quickly as he did and became frustrated when these discussions were extended. The clinician explained to this young man that all the questions and discussion necessary for these students to understand caused them to store the new information more effectively. On the other hand, he forgot the new problems because he had not worked hard to understand them. He was fooled by his own ability to conceptualize quickly and did not realize that he needed to do something to retain what he understood. Luckily, this student could reteach himself the math problems when he needed to but he seemed to appreciate that problems could result from his intolerance of old information particularly for subjects more challenging to him than math.

The student who likes a fast pace in class needs to be guided in planning short reviews that he/she can tolerate and using self-checking strategies to see if and when the old information has really been learned. Those who do not want extensive review of old information should be taught to ask specific questions that direct teachers to tell just what the student wants to know, without boring the student with unneeded information.

Students who prefer or need more old information should be guided in regularly previewing material for the next day's class in order to create an appropriate old/new balance for listening. Those college students who include a time for reconstructing and reviewing notes after class every day, are also advised to plan a regular time for previewing information before class, especially if the class is heavily loaded with new information and/or they have a need for extensive old information to guide their best processing.

When students understand the old/new balance, they can monitor their own learning more effectively and better understand their classmates' styles. Self-knowledge is not enough, however, and has to be supported by the learning of helpful, specific strategies (see Box 7–8). The previewing of tomorrow's work, daily reviewing of class notes and asking specific questions at the right times are good strategies for achieving an appropriate old–new information balance. The fast movers in learning may also use webbing to allow for quick previewing and reviewing. This same group may feel comfortable with key word notetaking and/or using drawing to translate information into a novel form that could also provide a review when needed. In any case, students need to know that everyone needs old and new information, that they may have a particular preference for balancing old and new information, that their teachers will also have styles reflecting their preferences and that there are strategies that take into account learning in view of the old–new balance.

BOX 7–8: *Ways to Balance Old–New Information*

1. Help students know their preferences
2. Discuss styles and strategies
3. For those who need *Old*:
   (a) Guide previewing and reviewing
   (b) Teach asking of specific questions
4. For those who need *New*:
   (a) Webbing with color coding
   (b) Key word notes
   (c) Drawing notes
   (d) Short reviews
   (e) Asking specific questions

Ask Questions

Asking questions (Figure 7–6) is an excellent learning strategy, but adolescents are not always adept at creating questions. It is critical to model, teach, help students generate a variety of question types, and guide practice at the various levels of questioning. Those who are not skilled at questioning will often limit themselves to the concrete questions that require simple answers (what, where, who). Pearson and Johnson, (1978) describe such questions whose answers are textually explicit, those one could point to in a text, as having a "right there" answer. These questions can be equated to Bloom's knowledge level, the lowest level of educational objectives (1965). These are the types of questions encountered often in the early grades, but they are not adequate to express all the inquiries of adolescents. Pearson and Johnson (1978) discussed more challenging questions whose answers are textually implicit and require that you infer the answer often by relating different facts in the text ("Think and search"). They described a third type of question that requires prior knowledge or an "internalized 'script'" in order to produce an "on my own" answer (Weaver, 1980, p. 236). Bloom's taxonomy (1965) has been suggested by many for helping students to expand their thinking in learning (see Nelson, 1998, p. 441) and to guide students in diversifying their question asking skill. Westby and Costlow (1991) provided examples of social studies questions matched to Bloom's levels of questioning. These questions can be used as models for students to match to other questions followed by discussion of how the matched questions are alike and for appreciation of the intent of the various questions.

Wiederhold (1997) provided examples for using Bloom's taxonomy applied to the Pledge of Allegiance with the lowest level, knowledge questions, asking the student to memorize and recite the pledge; the comprehension question asking for definitions of words; the application question requiring students to create a similar pledge to something they believe in; the analysis question requiring students to discuss the meaning of a phrase and to show its importance to the pledge; the synthesis question asking students to apply concepts in a new situation; the evaluation question asking for a judgment of the relative merits of the concepts and to tell how well the pledge achieves its goal. Students need many examples of the various levels of questions as models for learning, many opportunities to match questions by level, assignments requiring collection of various questions and then producing their own.

Questions for Warming-Up

One day Brent was asked to explain his homework assignment for an eleventh grade history class. He reported having to read "sections 7 and 8." I then asked Brent what the chapter was about and he did not know. So I turned to that chapter, showed Brent the title "World War II" and suggested he think of some questions about that topic to warm up for his reading. Brent looked surprised and quickly responded, "I don't ask the questions. You do." He clearly did not know that a learner asks questions in order to actively process new information, to decide on wheat from

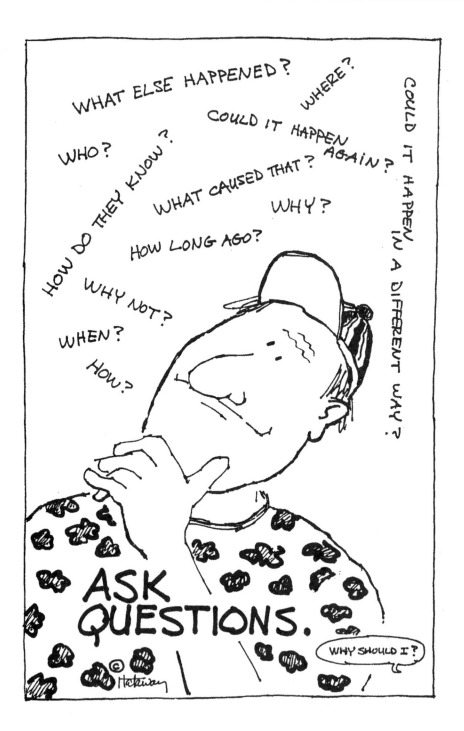

FIGURE 7-6

chaff, and so forth Before our next session, I prepared a skeletal web of Brent's chapter and used it to anchor Brent's attention visually as I gave a short overview of World War II. Surprisingly, he began spontaneously asking questions—not just simple questions but thoughtful, heuristic questions ("How come ... What if ... Why did ... "). It appeared that he could, under the right circumstances, ask very good questions and use this strategy in learning, but he was apparently unaware of the value of asking questions. Brent also did not know that he should familiarize himself with the topic before his daily reading—that he should know what he was reading about in order to fit details into an overall schema. He did not realize that an introduction to the topic and asking questions were active ways for processing new information.

Attending to Wrinkled Brows and Questions

It is helpful for instructors to identify those students presenting with a "wrinkled brow" showing their confusion who are obviously forming questions as they try to understand new information. Acknowledging students who are showing their learning in this way, helps students understand what "learning looks like," to create awareness of the internal confusion and accompanying questions that signal learning. Students need to understand that uncertainty and questioning symbolized by the "wrinkled brow" starts the learning process.

> If you have no questions—no wrinkled brow—then you will have no reason to pay close attention and if you don't pay attention you won't learn. Questions start the whole thing.

Brent and others who are struggling at learning often expect to automatically know answers and may be embarrassed to show that they have questions rather than quick answers. They need to know that all learners ask questions.

Young children are famous for the questions they ask that adults often cannot answer. ("Mommy, why don't the stars fall down?") Lindfors (1980) reported results of an informal observation of children's questions in the classroom. Student teachers were asked to stop periodically and write the questions they heard from students in the next several minutes. They noted that kindergartners and first graders asked challenging questions reflecting their natural curiosity about cause and effect, how things work and why. By third grade, however, students in this reported observation, asked mostly questions about procedure such as where to write their names, how long the paper had to be, when it was due, and so forth. If this is true and students begin to limit their intellectual curiosity by third grade, then it seems important to encourage questions more consciously and directly. Adolescents in particular need to be shown, guided and encouraged to notice the questions they have, to value those questions and use them as an important part of their learning.

Reserving Time for Questions in Class

How can we provide for and value questions within learning? It appears that educators need to plan for questions; build places into class routines for questions; show that questions are not just acceptable but needed for learning. Teachers also need to teach students how to ask a variety of questions.

Writing new topics on the board and collecting all the questions students can ask in warming up for a lesson communicates that teachers find questioning a viable learning strategy.

> Look at this topic. Ask all the questions that come to mind. Wrinkle your brow—then ask. I am not looking for any answers now—we just want as many questions as you can provide.

As a typical introduction to new lessons, this procedure can help students develop a list of questions to organize their attention to a new topic and practice asking those questions in the interest of learning. Students can be invited to ask questions before taking a pretest on a new topic. The teacher does not elaborate and simply provides exactly what is asked for, which seems a good way to stimulate further questions. The pretest is then given, a lecture/discussion ensues and then a post-test is given. This sequence can also structure the way chapters are studied in social studies and science with the reading of the chapter and discussion taking the place of a lecture.

Asking students to read or listen and generate possible test questions is an effective assignment. Dr. Sylvia Richardson (personal communication, 1975) told about a first grade teacher friend whose students were assigned the task of teaching their classmates. Parents were asked simply to provide the needed materials for the students' lecture/demonstrations. These young students explained many procedures including how to cook while camping. After each first grader was finished with his or her talk, the listening students asked questions. One of the favorite questions to ask of their 6-year-old peers was the following, "And how long have you been interested in this topic?" It appeared that these very young students were developing a repertoire of questions to ask at this time in this lesson. This kind of lesson with a regular question period can be continued through the grades and allow students to develop a wide variety of questions pertinent to and varied for different subjects and situations. Collecting helpful questions asked at these times, discussing what is effective about them, developing a rubric for asking questions and posting the rubric with many examples facilitates asking questions for those with language problems. The teacher needs to model a variety of question types also and, in some cases, the SLP may have to work individually with a student to practice higher level questions in a timely manner so they can utilize the time set aside for questions..

Having a regular time for questions will not seem novel to teachers who typically ask for questions following presentation of a new lesson or after giving oral directions. For those with language learning diffi-culties, however, it is not enough to merely say, "Does anyone have a question." We have to consider first whether the student knows he or she needs to ask; that is, are they actively monitoring their understand-ing or, like Jan in Chapter 4, nodding at the right times without realiz-ing that they are not processing. Then we have to find out if the student can formulate a question within the time limits appropriate to transi-tions in class. Teachers have to be sure that they are communicating that questions are valued. One math teacher, according to her students, said that it was important to ask questions before one became hopelessly confused. When someone asked a questions, however, this teacher's tone suggested that this was an unworthy question which, of course, squelched questions in this class. Therefore, we have to ensure that stu-dents feel safe asking questions, that they know when and how, and that they are taught to grow in the level of complexity of their questions.

Provoking Natural Questions

An activity that invariably provokes questions and shows students that asking questions is natural for them is writing an ambiguous statement on the board before class. (*"Do you know where he put it?"*) It is a rare student who does not wonder about what was lost, who put this object somewhere and where he put it. These kinds of ambiguous statements can provoke questions about short stories or novels or even expository chapters and serve as introductions to a lesson ("He was lucky to have lived during the Industrial Revolution and to see the changes that occurred in his country. This last invention determined his career for the rest of his life."). Questions provoked by this statement can be listed, answered and discussed in terms of their effectiveness. Students can discover which questions seem to evoke the most pertinent infor-mation, which questions seem to lead to other questions, and so forth.

Using Questions in Writing

Lucy Calkins (1983) described a report writing sequence in which stu-dents were assigned a topic, instructed to select an easy book on that subject, skimmed the book and brainstormed questions to start their thinking about the topic. This is a very practical way to elicit ques-tions—look through an easy book and wonder, then write all the ques-tions that come to mind. This way of warming up to the topic helps guide students' thinking before reading and gathering information for a writing assignment. Engaging in the question generating step in groups or learning pairs can help students develop more and varied questions for this step in the writing process.

Using Questions in Notetaking

Questions can be effective in notetaking also. Reading or listening and then creating possible test questions can cause good thinking about the information to be learned. This is also a good assignment to cause students to think about what a particular teacher has emphasized in discussions. Students can also be directed to rewrite their class notes in question form. Students can be given past tests in order to predict the questions that might be asked for a new chapter. They can study tests for several chapters on different topics and discuss the regularities. Asking students to study the teacher in class, the text book, their class notes or past tests and to formulate tests will be effective for processing information and for discovery of underlying patterns of questions.

Bloom's (1965) taxonomy of cognitive objectives has been frequently suggested for guiding students' development of increasingly more complex and abstract questions and for promoting development of thinking along a continuum (Wiederhold, 1997). Ideally, educators can provoke these questions with real experiences, such as science demonstrations or experiments; logic problems; reading incomplete accounts of accidents; telling stories that are interrupted and not finished as in the Harris Burdick story (Van Allsburg, 1984). Designing opportunities for evoking and capturing students' questions, then using these to show different types of questions is an ideal way to teach new language forms. There are many ways to provoke and promote questioning in learning, and this is a worthwhile goal if students are to appreciate and practice using questions as a necessary and regular part of the learning process. It is not enough to simply announce that asking questions is helpful. Questions must be planned for, modeled, and incorporated as an important element in learning. SLPs and teachers can collaborate to find effective ways for evoking a variety of questions asked at appropriate times within typical classroom activities (see Box 7–9).

BOX 7–9: *Ways to Promote Questions In Learning*

1. Provide questioning periods within learning scripts.
2. Show in your response, words and tone, that questions are valued.
3. Capture effective questions, analyze with group and develop a rubric for questions.
4. Model, search and collect, match, catch and elicit a variety of questions of varying levels of thinking.
5. Use questions for notetaking.
6. Use questioning for "warming up."
7. Use questions in writing assignments.

The Tutor Learns More Than the Tutee

Research on peer tutoring tells us that the tutor, the one helping a classmate learn, seems to learn more in this arrangement, than the tutee (see Figure 7–7), the student who needs the help (Gartner, 1993) although

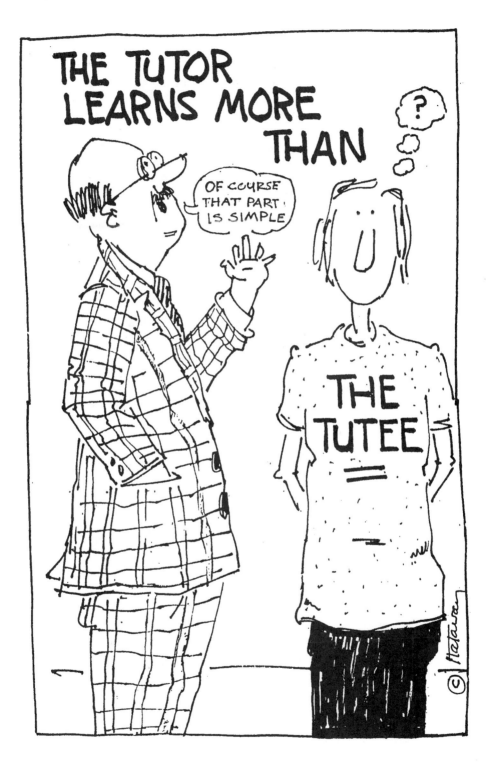

FIGURE 7-7

both students benefit from the tutoring in academic and social development (Cohen, Kulik & Kulik, 1982; Heden, 1987; Goodlad & Hirst, 1989; Greenwood, Delquadri & Hall, 1989; Benard, 1990; Swengel, 1991). The tutor's learning more is not surprising when one considers that the tutor must be active in explaining the concept or process in question. The tutor has to rephrase initial comments in response to the tutee or think of other ways to show rather than to tell a classmate what he or she is trying to teach. In trying to make something clear, the tutors test their own knowledge. They discover what they really understand and what they do not clearly understand.

This principle is regularly explained to students who are being tutored. They are advised to "Listen to what the tutor explains and then turn *yourself* into the tutor by re-explaining the information in your own words. Remember, the tutor learns more than the tutee, so give yourself that advantage. Become the tutor."

Modeling and Practicing the Tutor–Tutee Principle

"Because Wisdom cannot be told" (Gragg, 1940), we must engage students actively in listening and then paraphrasing explanations, followed by clarifications from the tutor and more paraphrasing ("Okay, see if I have this right. I think that you are saying this ... "). We often invite modeling and practice at home by having adolescents read their class notes aloud to a parent or friend who then "translates" the academic language into a more understandable paraphrase. After hearing this done many times, the students begin to read and paraphrase on their own. Many adolescents may need this kind of practice in order to restate what a tutor has taught. They might need the tutor to notice a wrinkled brow, encourage a specific question and then restate the information in a variety of ways, followed by the student's restating it, finally, in his or her own words.

The tutor–tutee practice can be completed in pairs with the two partners taking turns being tutors and tutees. This can be helpful for those students who overestimate their knowledge and do not study enough, for those students who are overly concerned and need reassurance even when they actually know the material, and for helping all students discover what they understand after a first presentation of new information. Distinguishing information that they might recognize on a multiple choice test as compared with that which they really understand well enough to explain in an essay answer will be obvious when students are challenged to explain what they know to a tutee.

Training Tutees to Become Tutors

Gartner (1993) reported that the Peer Research Laboratory at the City University of New York has been designing a model for using peer tutoring as an effective learning tool central to the instructional program rather than simply as a remedial strategy. In this model, students understand that when they are the tutees, they are being trained to later serve as tutors thus allowing them to acquire needed content in this paired learning model for a constructive purpose. The sixth graders, by Gartner's report, tutored second graders who then tutored younger students the following year. This approach seems appropriate for adolescents with special needs who may be motivated to learn in order to teach. This seems a good opportunity to direct attention to the content and the process of learning.

Provide Opportunities to Become Tutors

The easiest way to work this principle into classrooms is for teachers to regularly ask a student to explain the concept that has just been taught or the assignment that was given. Students will anticipate being a potential tutor at these junctures in class and may practice restating information. Training students to teach others within a variety of formats helps them learn in classrooms. Cooperative learning projects in which responsibility is divided among students who become knowledgeable about a topic and then teach others in the group, guide discussion, and create tests over the material provide effective learning, especially if the tutors are trained to ask for restatements of important points to allow their own tutees to become tutors. Palincsar and Brown (1984) describe reciprocal teaching in which the tutor (the teacher) first models predicting, summarizing the main idea, question generating and clarifying new vocabulary. Students in middle school are then chosen to become the teacher and proceed to facilitate comprehension in reading text using the reciprocal teaching approach. This is a good format for those with language and learning difficulties because the teacher shows how to guide the discussion and then supports learners as they try out the teaching. For instance, the teacher prompts the student to include the main idea only in the summary thereby teaching "wheat from chaff" and how to summarize. This is showing with telling and guided rehearsal.

Use Writing as a Tutor Activity

Harvey and Goudis (2000) guide students in selecting their topic of choice and creating "teaching books" (p. 127) as a vehicle for learning. This idea for younger students can be revised into "informative speeches" written by adolescents to teach others. When one considers that writing is an attempt to communicate ideas to others, this is a good way to become the tutor and solidify your own information. A summary of strategies to turn tutees into tutors is listed in Box 7–10.

BOX 7–10: *Ways to Turn Tutees into Tutors*

1. Regularly ask for paraphrases after lessons or directions.
2. Engage students in teaching within cooperative learning formats.
3. Model paraphrasing using class notes.
4. Engage in a training period as tutees who will become tutors.
5. Use the reciprocal teaching model.
6. Create teaching books.

Test Your Level of Knowing

Adolescents with learning problems often view homework as something to be finished but not necessarily understood. Students who are more successful realize, as they mature, that merely completing an assignment does not necessarily mean that they understand it, that they have been correct in their work, and/or that they have solidly stored the new information in long-term memory. All students need to know that testing their level of knowing is an important part of learning.

One middle school student arrived for a tutoring session and proudly announced that she had found and written the definitions for new vocabulary words. She was very pleased to be finished with a demanding task. Her tutor admired the several sheets of paper this assignment required and then commented, "This is a lot of work. Now, which words and definitions do you feel you know well, and which ones will require more review." The student looked surprised by this question, as though she had not considered checking her understanding and had assumed that completing the assignment was accomplishment enough.

Many students are angry when they have completed their homework and have studied for tests but receive a poor grade on the test. They seem to say that putting in the time should guarantee a good result. One has to sympathize because these students have done what they feel is required for school and they are confused when it doesn't work. They don't know that they need to test themselves to see how effective their work has been, to identify what they understand but may have to review to remember, and that which they clearly don't understand.

A very bright adolescent recently came for a consultation regarding his difficulties in learning foreign languages. He, his parents, and his instructors were baffled because this young man regularly completed homework on time and participated actively in class discussion, two ways that teachers know students are trying. He seemed to know the work as reflected in his comments in class but did poorly on tests.

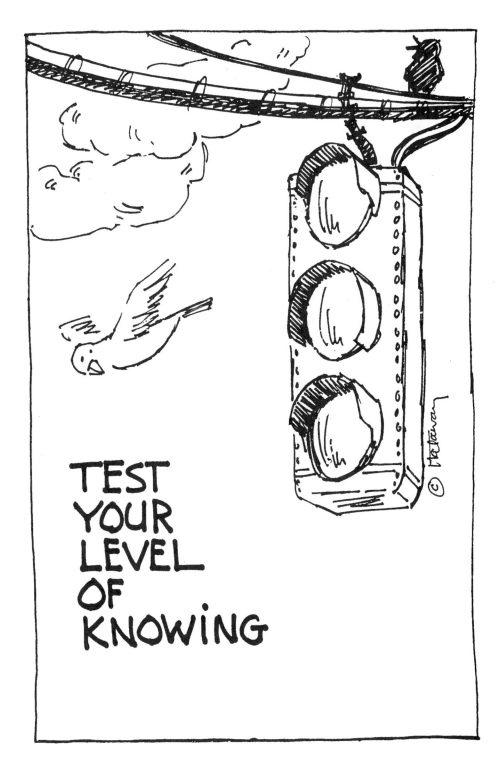

FIGURE 7-8

He explained the varied and active exercises in his language classes (translating back and forth between the two languages, making up sentences for new vocabulary, reading aloud from the text, etc). His studying at home, however, was very passive—he simply read over the material. Because he understood the work in class, he did not feel the necessity to study extensively at home and he applied this same approach successfully in studying for his other subjects. He did not appreciate that he apparently needed extra review in order to store what he had understood in his language classes. He never really checked what he understood and what he had stored for these classes. Adding a checking step to his studying—testing himself—seemed important for his foreign language classes. If this student found out what he knew and used some of the active in-class approaches at home to further study what he did not know, he could probably improve his test performance.

Checking for Red, Yellow and Green

It is helpful to sit shoulder-to-shoulder with adolescents to demonstrate ways to check their knowledge of what they have studied. We use a traffic light analogy to help students determine what they have learned and can tell or show quickly that they know (see Figure 7–8). The understood and well-stored information is categorized as "Green" knowledge, which means that it is clearly understood. (" You know this green information and are ready to go.") Perkins (1992) discussed the difference between possessing knowledge and understanding well enough to "to do things" with the knowledge (p. 76), which is consistent with our "green" knowledge as that which you thoroughly understand and can use. The concepts, facts or procedures that a student recognizes and seems to understand but cannot yet explain is deemed "Yellow" knowledge. Yellow can also be that which the student is learning, will probably be able to recognize in a multiple choice test, but cannot retrieve and utilize easily in an essay question. ("You are learning this material.") Having identified a concept as "yellow," students will need to show caution about this level of knowing. ("When it is yellow, you need to study it more thoroughly—review, explain, be able to demonstrate your knowing in a variety of ways. You are learning it."). They should understand that "yellow" knowledge shows potential, and they are on the verge of knowing that information. The remaining "Red" information is not understood yet and probably will not be recognized, recalled or explained well because the student has not yet learned it and will probably need help to do so. ("This is red. You have not yet begun to learn it and you may need to have someone else explain it or show you how to do it.")

As students begin to appreciate this traffic light analogy as a way of testing and labeling their level of knowing, instructors can collaborate with them to refine the categories. For instance, a student may have the information but seem tentative in discussing it, suggesting that it is "yellowish–green" or almost learned. They may recognize a concept but know little about it and this can be called "Reddish–yellow" or something that the student is ready to learn but has not really begun. This kind of discussion increases students' awareness of themselves as learners and suggests the amount of effort that must be expended in learning information at different levels. Many adolescents view all school learning as equal and do not categorize it in this way. They don't appreciate the "yellow" and simply value "green."

Checking by Parents

Adolescents sometimes ask their parents to quiz them as a way of testing, which is good, but parents often merely read the questions from a study guide and test memory rather than challenging the student to show understanding. Parents have to be guided to ask questions in a variety of ways or to check their child's understanding within a novel example or situation. They have to quiz in ways that ensure the child's knowing the information regardless of how the teacher asks for it. We often suggest that the student teach their parents the information first and then quiz them, utilizing the Tutor–Tutee principle along with self-testing in the process of explaining.

There are "understanding performances" suggested by Perkins (1992) that provide ways to test one's level of knowing: 1) explaining in your own words; 2) offering examples of the concept; 3) applying the knowledge in explaining something not yet studied; 4) justifying or defending the new concept with evidence; 5) comparing the new concept with something else; 6) exploring the relationship of the new information to the larger realm of knowledge in which it lies; and 7) telling the general principles that come from the new knowledge (the "So what"). (p. 77) Teachers can guide self-checking with follow-up assignments using these activities. Instead of the usual "going over last night's assignment" in a simple rehashing, it may be helpful to have students explain (become the tutor), to compare with another topic or project, prove the information with example, place the new information in the context of the overall class subject, science, social studies, and so forth.

Recognizing What You Do Not Understand

I often ask students to repeat a Japanese greeting "Listen as I say a phrase and then I want you to repeat it : 'Ohiogazeimus'" They can usually repeat this phrase without difficulty showing their ability to remember something they do not understand, which is dangerous in studying. ("You did well, but what good did that do for you to be able to say that? Do you understand what you said? No? I didn't think so.") This phrase then serves as a way to label, for English-speaking students, that which they can repeat but do not really understand. For instance, if a student reads class notes aloud but cannot rephrase those notes in his or her own words, this is labeled an "Ohiogazeimus." ("You certainly recalled what was said in the book but I'm wondering if this is an 'Ohiogazeimus' for you. Can you explain it another way?") A different word or even a nonsense word can be used in the same way to represent information a student can read and recall but does not understand well enough to restate. Having a term for memorizing without understanding directs students to test their real understanding in learning and contrast it with mere memorizing.

Students who begin to accurately judge what they know well, know partially, or do not know at all have potential for taking control of their learning and improving their school performance. They find out what they merely need to study more on their own as compared with when they need help to really understand. In collaborating with adolescents who are struggling in school, it is important to help them view self-assessment as a strength ("You will have more potential as a learner if you become an expert on what you know and don't know. Even when you are doing badly in a subject, your knowing exactly what you need to study differently or harder will help you improve.") and to guide regular practice to evaluate their own knowledge. Because of time constraints, adults often continue to check the students' level of knowing. Since the arrows in these kinds of teaching–learning transactions start and end with the teacher (see Chapter 2), the students may not take over the job of evaluating their own learning.

Recently a math tutor was asked to help a high school junior complete a correspondence course to satisfy a math requirement. The tutor was frustrated because this student seemed to understand concepts or processes in individual lessons but not to retain them. She mailed lessons without checking them over and seemed intent only on finishing the course. She didn't seem aware that, without really understanding the math required in each completed lesson, she could not pass the final exam. Having identified this problem the tutor decided on the following plan: to ask her student to first read over a review and predict how well she knew the material by marking each problem with a green, yellow or red dot. The student would then complete the review test that would be graded by the tutor. The student could note the accuracy of her self-assessment (the colored dots vs. final grading). The tutor felt that increasing the student's self-knowledge would be as important as her math ability, especially in determining what and how much to study. Students such as this young lady can be required to judge their knowledge by placing such dots beside test questions. Teachers can reward them for self-knowledge with extra points but require that they learn the red and yellow answers later. Those who are consistently accurate on dotting test answers but don't improve may need to apply this same dot system to homework assignments, to design further active study and to compare their study dots with later test dots to assess their self-testing in studying.

Just like Brent (see Asking Questions above) who thought that he was not the one who asked the questions, this math student may have assumed that it was the teachers and parents who would monitor her strengths and weaknesses and take appropriate action rather than her taking over the assessing of her own learning needs. Some students persist in this view of learning as something owned by teachers. One wonders if the typical comment of instructors that a student "worked really well for me today" perpetuates this dependence on teachers as responsible for the learning.

Applying the "Test your level of knowing" principle consistently and accurately seems appropriate for transferring the ownership of their learning to all students, but it is especially critical for students in transition to college or work. With well-established, ongoing self-evaluation, they will know their strengths and weaknesses that can guide their problem solving and allow them to advocate more intelligently for appropriate help in learning and on the job. Without self-testing, students will not know what they need in different situations (see Box 7–11).

BOX 7–11: *Ways to Encourage Self-testing*

    1. Require that students label homework assignments as Red-Yellow-Green.

    2. Model and practice paraphrasing (Ohiogazeimus).

    3. Ask students to predict their knowledge of practice tests.

    4. Require more than just telling (comparing, justifying, applying, etc.).

    5. Use the "dot" system on tests and reward self-knowledge.

Understand the Topic Versus the Point

Adolescents seem confused about the difference between the topic, that is, what a reading passage, a lecture, a discussion or a writing piece of their own, a statement or question is *about* as contrasted with what is *being said about the topic at hand,* that is, the point that is being made. Although the concept of the main idea is introduced early in elementary school, it continues to be difficult for many students to determine the main idea in their reading (Bauman, 1983). When asked to tell about a paragraph they have read, some students offer terms or short phrases that seem to be topics rather than to explain the point of the passage. When students fail to write in complete sentences this can reflect a confusion about topics and points to be made about a topic. Adolescents' writing can have limited shape and consist of a list of facts relevant to the topic with no unifying theme or main idea. When asked to generate ideas for writing, many students produce topic ideas (Rap) but do not go further to refine their topic into a possible point

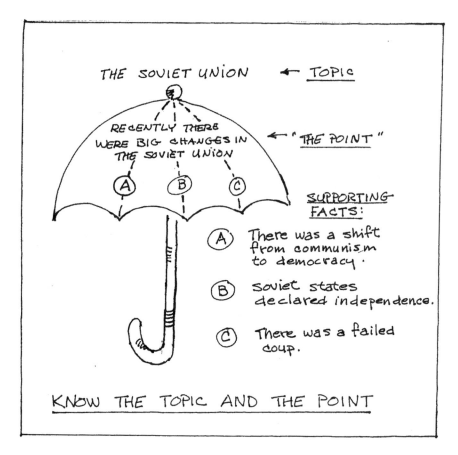

FIGURE 7-9

(There are Rappers who are not violent.) that would help them organize their thinking beyond a list of sentences about that topic.

Writing Around a Topic

Graves (1983) describes the early writings of children. Rather than organizing their information into a narrative form or even imposing a chronologic order, their statements seem to simply "swirl around one topic" (p. 194). Sometimes one sentence leads to another and then a third sentence addresses a slightly different aspect of the topic. There is a clear focus on each thought but without a tying together with a main idea. Early writing often progresses to an organization that places events in time and the writer seems to arrive at the central action only by starting from home in the early part of the day and describing all events as they occurred, with somewhat equal emphasis on each event. Graves calls this organization a "bed to bed" story (p. 156) and it is often signaled by the "and then" connector, more advanced than using simply "and," and reflects equal value of sentences but adds the importance of time order. One can see these same characteristics in adolescents' writing when they are struggling with language development in general and/or if they have written very little and are really beginning writers. In all these instances, the young writers seem keenly aware of the topic but not the need to make a particular point about the topic. We need to help them stop "swirling" in favor of making a point. Williams (1985) suggested that appreciation of the main idea "rests strongly on categorization and classification skills" (p. 22) and she described a teaching procedure that elicited these basic skills using familiar content first. She asked students to identify the "general topic" (What is the paragraph about?) and then to focus on the main idea as the "specific topic" (What does the paragraph tell about squirrels?) (van Dijk, 1980).

Understanding Topic–Point in Sentences

In our work to help students clearly understand questions, we ask them to identify the topic (What is this question about?), the fact that gets at the point of the question (What fact do you learn about that topic, just from reading this question?) and the direction inherent in the question (What must you do to answer the question?). Just as they have difficulty identifying main ideas in longer passages, students seem to have difficulty uncovering the facts in this process of dissecting a question. They often produce a phrase or topic rather than a fact in answer to the second question suggesting, again, a confusion between topic and comment or point. It is interesting that when students seem to have misread a test question, their answer usually addresses the correct topic but misses the point or fact in the question.

Focusing on Points

One student copied cause–effect statements provided by the teacher to guide students' preparation for a test about the Revolutionary War. A short discussion showed that this student did have even a basic understanding of the topic, the Revolutionary War, and yet she seemed ready to memorize isolated statements without appreciation for their meaning.

Addressing Topic and Point in Conversation

In casual conversations, adolescents seem to address the topic and to, naturally, make a specific point about that topic—they know what they are talking about and what particular point they want to make. If they are bored by someone who seems to be rambling, it is not unusual for an adolescent to say, "So what is your point?" If they enter an ongoing conversation or come in late in watching a TV show, most adolescents will ask about the topic in order to understand, suggesting an intuitive appreciation for topic as context for comprehension. In their reading and writing, however, these same youngsters may not stop to be sure they have the topic in mind to guide their processing of points to be made.

Presuming Topic–Point Understanding

The principle of understanding and clearly separating the topic and comment or point seems so self-evident that it is presumed by educators. Although they introduce topics before exploring the points to be made about them, they often do not remind students to check to see if they are aware of the connections between points to be made and the topic. The suggestions under the warm-up principle are designed to establish the topic solidly as a base for understanding expository texts or fiction to be read. The various ways to introduce the topic can be effective, but students need to be able to tell and show, periodically, knowledge of what is being discussed and what is being said about this topic—to be very clear on the forest versus the trees in each discussion. They need to understand that an author has a purpose, an axe to grind about a topic and one needs to find the point that is being made.

Establishing Topic and Point in Expository Chapters

In reading expository chapters, previewing the whole chapter first is a way to introduce and familiarize students with the topic, before each section of the chapter is read. After each paragraph in a section, students can be guided to ask two questions similar to those asked by Williams (1985): "What is this paragraph about? (The topic of the paragraph). What point is being made in this paragraph about this topic?" After hearing teachers and other students model the reading of paragraphs in this way, at risk students may better appreciate the difference between the topic and the point of each paragraph, that all the paragraphs under a subtitle have the same topic but a different point, and that every paragraph exists to make a point.

Using An Umbrella Analogy

We have used an umbrella to show the hierarchical-meaning relationships in paragraphs (see Figure 7–9). The topic of each paragraph is written over the knob at the end of the umbrella and the point or main idea is written along the surface of the opened umbrella. The facts or examples that support the point being made are represented by the umbrella's spokes. These levels of meaning need to be shown and reviewed often to tie the meaning of individual facts or examples to the main points they illustrate under a subtopic which is a part of the overall topic or chapter title. Instructors can use the umbrella illustration to place students' comments under the topic showing main idea or supporting comments.

Constructing and Reconstructing Webs

Constructing a web in the previewing of chapters, then as the chapter is read and discussed, adding main points under subtitles on the web, followed by supporting examples or facts, is another way to help students see these relationships. This visual representation or the umbrella illustration can remind teachers to continue to comment on the relationships among levels of information as they are building meaning within the study of a chapter. Presenting a blank version of the initial web with spaces for topic and subtopics can guide the review and/or self-testing of students' recall of information for a chapter or unit of study. In small groups students, can be challenged to fill out and explain the relationships of ideas on the web with reminders to ask the topic–point questions (What was this part about? What were the points made in each paragraph? What support was there for the points?). They can then test their recall by comparing their reconstructed web with the one completed during the study of the chapter in class. This reconstructing of webs can be presented as a self-test for each student with the challenge to note what they omitted in their reconstruction and to devise better ways to learn that information. This web constructing–reconstructing strategy seems a good scaffold for learning topic–point relationships.

Going from Topic to Comment

Authors of textbooks often provide key words or phrases in the review sections at the end of a chapter or in bold print within the chapter. These words and phrases represent topics about which students must construct comments or full sentences in order to understand. An effective exercise for homework is to ask students to write fact statements about each key word or to identify the important topics (wheat) presented in the chapter and then make comments about them. In a Section Assessment section in one high school text (Danzer et al., 1998), in an exercise subtitled, "Analyzing," students are asked a question: "What factors do you think contributed to the thriving trade system that flourished in West Africa? Use evidence from the text to support your response." They then are provided key phrases to "think about" including "geographic location and features, the kinds of goods exchanged and the societies that emerged in West Africa." (p. 19). This is a wonderful curriculum for modeling the identifying of the larger topic (Thriving trade system in West Africa) and the point made about that topic found in the question provided ("There are factors that contribute to the thriving trade system that flourished in West Africa.") with awareness of the direction within the question ("I must find those factors and use evidence from my reading to support my answer."). These students can be shown how to note the topics in the "think about" section, to read and generate points about each topic. In so doing, they will be clear on what they are talking about (topics) as contrasted with the point being made about each topic.

Generating Points

Adult collaborators can write a topic and ask students in a group to simply write a sentence about that topic. For instance, one can write "Coffee" and elicit various comments: "Coffee smells better to me than it tastes ... Hosts and Hostesses assume all people drink coffee ... The new flavored coffees do not seem like real coffee ... " Any one of these points can be elaborated into a paragraph that can then be shown on the umbrella illustration with the topic on top (Coffee), the point written across the open umbrella and the supporting statements leading to the points written on the spokes. Because the topic is constant and the points are different in this exercise, the difference between these levels of language can be made clear (see Box 7–12).

BOX 7–12: *Ways to Contrast Topic and Point*

1. Ask about the topic and the point in discussions, reading, and writing.
2. Identify topic and point in paragraphs, statements, and questions.
3. Show topic–point relationships in umbrella illustrations and webs.
4. Generate points around the same topic.

Solve Problems

A mother explained that her daughter, Kathy, had an assignment book but often left it at school. This led to a discussion of possible plans for remembering to bring the assignment book home after school. The mother then asked, "But what if Kathy is sure she has it, sees no reason to check, and then comes home without it?" This was a fair question and presented another problem that required a revision of the original plan to ensure that Kathy actually saw the assignment book in her bag before she left for home.

Viewing Problem Solving as Ongoing

It was important, in this effort, for Kathy and her mother to understand that problem solving is ongoing. This mother was distraught about her daughter's difficulties and seemed convinced that there would be one problem after another. She seemed to want one solution that would cover all the school organization, language and learning problems. She had to appreciate that if the first plan does not work, one always has to determine the new problem and revise that plan. She had to understand that she and her daughter would have to persist in problem solving until the assignment book was consistently brought home and this particular problem was solved. The problem solving principle had to be invoked and presented in the most basic way using the picture on the poster to show that problem solving rarely stops and that one simply continues to identify each new problem very clearly, to make a plan, try it out and keep revising the plan until it works (see Figure 7–10). Then one begins on another problem area.

The next problem posed by this mother was that her daughter often started her homework without understanding the assignment. Kathy's teacher reported the same impulsive behavior in school. The suggested plan for this problem added a step in the regular study routine. Kathy was required to first explain her understanding of the homework assignment and then read and explain the directions to her mother and decide if her predictions were correct. The mother clarified as needed; Kathy explained what she then understood and proceeded to do the work. If Kathy protested about this plan after trying it at home, she was to suggest her own modifications with the understanding that a check of her homework for a week would show whether her plan was working. The mother, in this case, had forgotten two appointments during our collaboration, and it was suggested that these were good examples for discussing everybody's need for problem solving. She could explain her plan for remembering appointments in the future to show her daughter that she was working on her own specific problems.

As this example shows, it is necessary to emphasize problem solving with parents and students. It is a working principle applicable to schoolwork. Although most families problem solve naturally to negotiate busy, complicated lives, they need to engage in conscious and regular problem solving with their children regarding homework or school.

Understanding the Diagnostic Process as Problem Solving

Using the problem solving principle also helps parents understand the diagnostic process when they seek help. The author regularly asks parents who call requesting testing, "What question are we trying to answer with testing?" which helps clarify problems to be addressed. Kathy's mother wanted to know whether her daughter had a significant school learning problem, and to clearly understand her strengths and weaknesses. She provided observations that contributed significantly to identifying problems in the diagnostic process. She identified patterns in her daughter's studying. For instance, the mother said her daughter seemed to memorize information easily but could not then answer test questions. She said that her daughter could read words

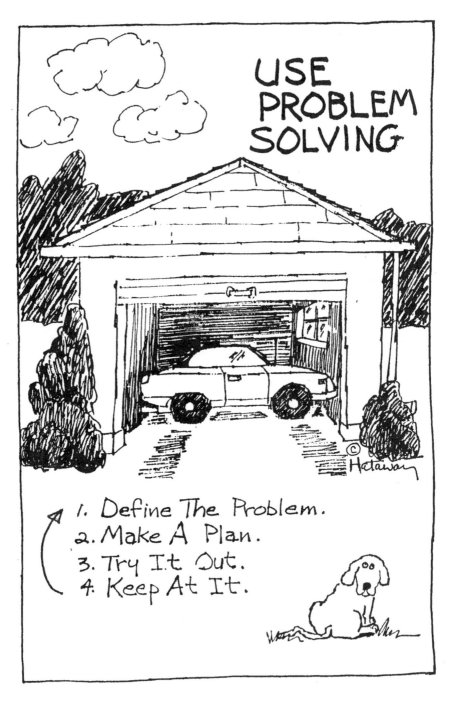

FIGURE 7-10

well but did not know what she had read and that she seemed to need to be re-taught what she should have learned at school. In spite of continuing difficulties in school, however, the mother reported that her daughter seemed overconfident about what she thought she knew and did not ask questions. These observations, taken with the test results, showed a pattern of strength in expressive, conversational skills. Kathy showed below average receptive language skills, good word reading and spelling skills, but poor oral and reading comprehension. Her impulsive decisions in testing suggested a lack of appreciation for the need to reflect on harder tasks consistent with the reports of overestimating her understanding of lessons. The final pattern showing stronger surface skills compared with the weaker comprehension and limited self-knowledge or self-testing seemed clear.

The next step in problem solving with this family was to make plans to influence Kathy's comprehension of school lessons and self-testing. The parents, school, and student would contribute to devising and implementing plans, evaluating and making revisions as needed. The problem solving principle was illustrated in this evaluation/collaboration process.

Identifying Problems and Accompanying Feelings

Another adolescent girl, Anne, with a similar pattern of weak organization for school, was engaged in learning the Number–Rhyme system (Buzan, 1974) for recalling the first 10 presidents in order. She was to learn 10 object words that rhymed with the numbers from 1 to 10 (one–bun, two–shoe, etc.) then associate each president's name with the appropriate number–rhyme word to facilitate recall of the presidents' names in the order in which they served. The problem solving principle was invoked when Anne could not remember the eight–gate hook. The plan was to create a mental picture with exaggerated associations to ensure her remembering this hook on the next trial. Anne drew a picture and the SLP added exaggerated characteristics associating a "gate" with the number 8. In the next recall trial, Anne remembered the hook. Anne was delighted to have this success in a learning activity and that was good, but it was important to discuss what had happened in terms of problem solving—to direct her attention to the process of identifying the problem, making a plan, trying it out and then using the plan. This activity also supplied opportunities to evaluate plans. When Anne made an association between the sixth president, John Quincy Adams, and the sixth hook (sticks), her association did not prevent her confusing this president with his father, John Adams, the second president. Anne revised her plan to make a foolproof connection between "sticks" and John Quincy Adams and the second plan worked. She did not confuse the two in her recall. Anne was so caught up with the fun of creating absurd, memorable association pictures and with her success in the activity that it seemed critical to discuss what had transpired. This discussion or "meta" step would better ensure that Anne understood the problem solving that had occurred. We discussed how she felt when she could not remember one of the items and that she might have stopped problem solving at that point because she felt embarrassed and "dumb" but that we had persisted in revising the plan until it worked. We continued in this exercise and Anne was able to recall all the presidents but two. We discussed the need to skip difficult items in tasks such as these or on tests, rather than to let her feelings interfere and cause her to miss points for those she knew.

Providing Time for and Discussion of Problem Solving in Class

In most learning experiences, there are instances where problem solving is necessary and students who appreciate this become creative in the solutions or plans they devise. Providing a time to specifically identify and discuss problems associated with school assignments allows students to accept problem solving as a respected part of learning first. A second advantage for focusing directly on problems in learning is that students gain skill in explaining their strategies for solving problems. Hearing other students helps other students learn how to discuss problems and it provides a variety of new strategies to guide plans for school problem solving (see Box 7–13). Stretching students' attention beyond simply completing homework to reflection on the process is productive. Regularly engaging groups of students in post-mortem discussions of problems and solutions also shows less successful students that problems occur for everyone—even those who seem to be more facile in their learning; that the problem solving principle is not just for problem learners. How effective it would be, for instance, for students to be engaged in writing a trial term paper before attempting one on their own. Students walked through the writing process can

---

BOX 7–13: *Ways to Promote Problem Solving in Learning*

1. Regularly include discussion of problems in homework assignments.
2. Model and practice whole or small group walk–throughs of difficult assignments (term papers) to identify problems and solutions.
3. Discuss the impact of feelings that stops problem solving.
4. Identify specific problems within usual assignments and teach/practice strategies.
5. Demonstrate so parents and students understand that problem solving is ongoing.
6. Challenge students to predict needed principles for specific assignments.

identify problems and solutions, discuss them in groups and work in whole groups which can provide a model for writing their individual term papers. Having the poster available allows teachers and students to remember to use and discuss problem solving as a regular part of learning.

■ SUMMARY

This chapter has presented ten principles for guiding learning and increasing adolescents' awareness of learning processes and of themselves as learners. The "warm-up" principles stresses the necessary "priming" or familiarizing oneself with the overall topic as a preparation for listening, reading or writing. Knowing that "there's more than one way to skin a cat" encourages students to explore optional strategies for understanding and proceeding within a learning task rather than assuming that there is one answer. The third principle, "wheat from chaff," makes clear that one must prioritize attention to the important information in listening, reading and writing. The "what—so what?" principle highlights the need to ask why you are learning something—to understand not just isolated facts but to tie pieces of information to the topic, to other facts being presented and to the purpose for learning each fact. Appreciation of the "old–new balance" is necessary for best attention and learning and underscores the value of "warming up" and "solving problems" when you are bored with too much old information and may miss a transition to something new. "Ask questions" is a principle invoked to encourage active processing of information and to reinforce the importance of understanding rather just accepting and memorizing what is going on in schoolwork. It is necessary to teach many students how to ask questions, to value questions as an important part of learning and to plan regular opportunities for questioning. Talking about and demonstrating the "tutor–tutee" principle shows students the importance of restating information in their own words. "Test your level of knowing" actively promotes students' knowing their own strengths and weaknesses and not assuming that simply finishing homework ensures that they really understand it. Appreciating the distinction of "topic versus point" can ensure more effective processing of paragraphs, questions and sentences and provides a good way for students to evaluate the clarity of their own writing. Finally, the "solve problems" principle underscores the need to identify problems, make plans, evaluate and revise those plans, then make each plan a habit. Discussion focused on the need for ongoing problem solving and the possible interference of emotions in the problem solving process.

It is productive to notice and note how adolescents naturally apply these learning principles in their own lives. The real world examples lay the groundwork for introducing each principle by name and with a visual representation. Once established as shared concepts that find their origins in the real life of adolescents, these principles can be invoked for conscious use within school assignments. The educator in this collaboration should continue to "catch" students applying these principles naturally, which enhances awareness of natural learning abilities; to teach and guide conscious practice of the principles within school assignments; and to challenge students to independently identify those principles critical to specific assignments and/or those which have general value in school. These principles can be used as a tool for students to identify and produce "quality work" (Glasser, 1993b).

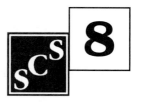

Language Strategies for Extended Discourse

The academic language confronting adolescents as they progress in school is different from that of conversation and many students are not prepared for this kind of discourse. They often cannot adequately understand the language of class discussion or their textbooks. Some students' language problems have been previously identified because of oral language delays and these students will, undoubtedly, have difficulty with academic language. There are also those who may have passed the language tests typically given by speech-language pathologists and never qualified for language intervention. There may be a third group whose speech was clear, who could engage adequately in short interchanges and/or kept a low profile in classes saying very little so they might never have been identified as having communication insufficiencies. However, the language of the classrooms beginning in fourth grade and continuing through high school and college requires more than the short interchanges of conversation and these last two groups will be confronted with academic language they cannot manage. An adolescent can remain in a conversation with peers for a long time by periodically saying, "Cool," but will need decidedly more skill to participate effectively in class discussions or to read an expository text. Many adolescents will need to be taught how to manage this kind of language.

■□ CONTRASTING BICS AND CALPS

Cummins (1981) noted the contrast between BICS and CALPS. BICS stands for *Basic Interactional Conversational Skills* and is what our language tests typically address. CALPS stands for *Cognitive Academic Language Proficiency Skills* for which casual conversation does not prepare us. This kind of language is different from conversation, requires more effort and is particularly challenging for those with language learning problems. Cummins discusses BICS versus CALPS in reference to those learning a second language and warns that being able to manage in a conversation may not ensure success in classrooms. There are implications in the BICS–CALPS contrast for many students for whom the academic language is akin to a foreign language even though they are native English speakers. As these students move to higher grades the demands for language processing increase and they must learn to listen, read and produce this new kind of language. Luetke-Stahlman (1998), writing with hearing impaired students in mind, used the Cummins model to show a continuum of cognitive demands in language proceeding from easy information to difficult information. Intersecting this cognitive dimension in the model, there is also a continuum of contextual support from information embedded in a supportive context. to information presented within a very reduced level of context. Tasks involving BICS can be conceptualized as those that are "cognitively-undemanding" (Luetke-Stahlman p. 67), include familiar ideas and vocabulary in familiar, informal, sometimes routine exchanges. Tasks requiring CALPS, on the other hand, are represented as those that are cognitively demanding, lack social situational cues and may vary in contextual support for understanding. CALPS are considered essential for school learning, for evaluating information in terms of relationships, inferences, and conclusions, for having analytical discussions, for understanding complex narratives and expository text, for evaluating ideas and explaining information in a formal way (Chamot, 1981). Without skills for academic language, students are limited in their potential as thinkers and students.

■□ IDENTIFYING THOSE AT RISK

Many students' conversational limitations are identified early and addressed within speech language therapy. There are also those with impoverished oral language skills caused by limited experience and these students are sometimes supported because of their lack of readiness for school. Students with early language problems are at even greater risk when the language demands increase in school. As noted above there are also students who fare well in the short interchanges of conversation but are not ready for the demands of higher level, formal language and may go unnoticed until they confront the language of expository texts or classroom lectures. Teachers, parents and even the students themselves may not realize that they have a language problem because their speech is usually clear and they speak in appropriate basic sentences adequate for conversation. There is, however, a need for direct teaching for the level and style presented by CALPS and for guided practice including, at the very least, a focus on strategies for reading expository chapters, for comprehending and producing paragraphs, for processing complex statements and questions and for managing new and challenging vocabulary. This chapter will present strategies for these language challenges.

■□ IDENTIFYING THE LANGUAGE CHALLENGES OF EXPOSITORY TEXT

Students are presented with increasingly abstract and unfamiliar topics as they progress in school. Naturally, they should encounter new topics because they are learning but to maintain a proper old–new balance, some part of the task has to be familiar or easy. Unfortunately these unfamiliar topics are discussed within complex language forms that are also unfamiliar. Westby (1985), discussed the progression of language from the easiest conversational level to the more challenging language of fiction through the most challenging language of exposition. Sentences become longer and more complex in fiction but the topics usually include those of real life and the focus is on people. The reader brings experience from the real world that is relevant in reading fiction. Fiction also has a "strong script" (Perera, 1986) that carries us along and, after the basic story is introduced, it becomes easier to understand. This is not so with nonfiction. Each part of an expository chapter can require equal effort in processing the information. The chapter does not become easier near the end. Expository text is often far removed from the topics and language of conversation; is less personal than fiction; provides few direct quotes; replaces personal pronouns with the impersonal "it" or "they" (referring to objects); and the agents of the action are often not stated explicitly. Perera provides an extreme example of an expository sentence that seems contrived to *not* include the agent: "During the seventeenth century the roads became a little straighter." (p. 55)

Discourse in expository test is organized by higher level connector words such as "nevertheless, similarly, heretofore, whereas ... " that are unlike the connector words that many adolescents would find familiar: "first, then, also, finally, so." Passages are less cohesive when students are unsure of how thoughts are connected. Students are presented with many more new concepts in nonfiction and these concepts are often not repeated, which requires conscious information processing. In expository text, students confront many different and new kinds of discourse. Conversation also presents a variety of kinds of discourse but they are familiar and the language is not so complicated. Stories are often organized in time which is easier to follow than the topical organization of expository texts. Sentences are more complex in academic texts, a style which is inappropriate in conversation so students have usually had less experience in hearing or reading this kind of language. They are often unprepared for the long clauses that interrupt the basic sentence in nonfiction, for instance: "The agouti, a very nervous 20 inch, 6 pound rodent that lives in South America, can leap twenty feet from a sitting position." (Perera, 1986, p.58) Students are regularly advised to make their own writing more clear by using action verbs, but expository texts written for students 9–14 years of age often are written in passive tense and one has to reconstruct the agent–action–object sequence. The complex nouns phrases and verb phrases can be very difficult to follow: "The few which are large enough to survive the fall through the air and actually reach the ground are called meteorites." (Perera, p. 61)

■□ KEEPING ADOLESCENTS IN THE "LITERACY CLUB"

Smith (1988) admonished us to keep students in the "Literacy Club" and, as literacy includes processing of oral and written language, this becomes important as students are confronted with a new and difficult kind of literacy. We have to keep adolescents in the Literacy Club so they can continue to enjoy the advantages that higher language provides. Conscious planning for specific kinds of help may be necessary.

Both those who reach adolescence with known oral language problems and those for whom it is extended discourse that causes the problem, language help is necessary. If we do not identify this as a problem and address it, then we will continue to simply screen out those without natural talent in higher level language.

Discussion thus far has been focused on those students who are at risk for language processing and the extra stress placed on them by higher-level language, but Tonjes (1986) makes a different point. She says that we must consider teaching most students to make the leap to "study-reading" and thinking skills required as they advance in school; that study reading is related to cognitive thought and they might not have been ready to learn this kind of language processing earlier.

■□ READING EXPOSITORY CHAPTERS

The "warm-up" information presented earlier is important for providing background information to counteract the difficulties presented by unfamiliar topics. Teachers need to find out through prereading discussion if students have the requisite background information and, if not, to provide it as a base for understanding new information. Evoking related real world experience with many examples can help students personalize the material and increase their motivation to read. (Tonjes 1986). We need to ensure a supportive meaning context when students are confronted with expository tasks and if we do, they will be better able to manage difficult material.

Adolescents who arrive for classes or for diagnostic testing in our Center rarely have a conscious strategy for reading their textbooks. They typically open the text to the first page of the chapter and begin to read—not a good formula for comprehension. To improve their school performance, adolescents need a different way to read a chapter.

Strategies pertinent to reading chapters have been introduced earlier in this book (DRTA, SQ3R, etc.). Many teachers recognize the SQ3R approach, for instance, as something they have heard about but have never really used themselves nor have they directed their students to use it.

Presenting and Practicing "How to Read a Chapter"

We have been modifying these approaches with our How To Read A Chapter lessons for adolescents in an effort to provide a functional process which students might be willing to use (see Box 8–1). Before introducing this process, it may be effective for a class to complete a chapter in their usual way and to be tested as usual with the teacher recording the mean score as a base line. Then the teacher can model/teach the new process for reading a chapter in a walk-through whole class experience followed by discussion and students' explaining the process in their own words to ensure understanding. Students could then be tested on this walk-through chapter, the mean test score figured for this chapter compared to that of the prior chapter. Adolescents are skeptical and may be motivated by improvement shown in scores.

BOX 8–1: *How to Read a Chapter*

  1. Read the **title** and think (What do I know or what can I guess about this?)

     Now you have a brain file ready for information.

  2. **Skim** the chapter and **make a web** with the title in the middle and the subtitles around the web.

     Now you have a picture of the overall topic and the parts.

  3. Read the **summary,** if there is one (or the main idea and study questions at the beginning of the chapter) and then guess where facts would fit on your web. Write **key words** or fact statements under subtitles.

     Now you have a fatter file and a more complete web.
     You are ready to read.

     (continued)

BOX 8–1: *(continued)*

  4. **Read each section** of the chapter in this way. Read the subtitle, think, read each paragraph and stop to ask yourself (What is this about? What point are they making about that subject?) **Write the important point** for each paragraph. Put it on your web.

  Now you have read each section and have notes for studying.

Of course, just walking students through this chapter reading strategy in a group may not ensure that individual students will use it. A second phase might place students in pairs to study the next chapter with the challenge to create a web similar to that of the teacher to be shown later for comparison and discussion of what was chosen and why. A third chapter can be completed repeating this paired learning activity with the students discussing what they have included and/or omitted, using the teachers completed web as their standard. The next chapter can be studied independently with students' checking their own webs with the teacher's and, again, discussing differences in order to understand "what" was included and why ("so what?"). Finally, the students are asked to read their chapter independently using the outline they have learned without the backup of the teacher's web.

Varying the Approach to Reading Chapters

There are variations on this way of reading and studying a chapter. Sometimes the previewing is shortened to simply constructing a web based on the outline of the chapter shown in the Table of Contents, then reading the summary or final chapter questions before reading. Having a large web of the chapter constructed with the group and assigning small groups to study subsections and create mini-webs can be followed by students fanning out to become tutors using the mini-web from their groups to teach others.

Another variation asks the students in groups to generate vocabulary lists based on reading the title only, then the subtitles, then the summary. Groups compare their vocabulary lists as a warm-up with discussion of why they included words in their lists and how the words are associated with the topic. Then students read the chapter, adding vocabulary to their lists as needed. The vocabulary words can be put on a web under appropriate subtitles or just left in a list. Finally at the end of the chapter reading, the list of words are grouped and students create statements for each group of words. Whatever approach to reading a chapter, creating a web showing the title and subtitles seems helpful in establishing a context which shows visually the relationship of ideas to the subtitles and title.

Reading Fiction

English teachers seem to thoroughly discuss fiction and to give specific outlines for book reports or for writing assignments that direct students to the "wheat" as they read. For many years it seemed unnecessary, then, to help students comprehend the fiction they read so we focused more on expository texts. We began to get complaints from adolescents with language problems, however, that they were having problems in comprehending the fiction that was assigned. Our work on reading and understanding expository text reading was expanded to include fiction with these students. We have begun by guiding these students' "warm-up" for reading fiction. We first model reading a book aloud to the group, stopping periodically to tell what we know. We read until we have a basic understanding, a mental file, that can guide our comprehension as we read further. We have built a context for further reading and understanding. The students are asked to select a novel or short story; to read and find the earliest place in the text where they can form a tentative mental file and can make a good guess at these questions:

> Who are the characters? What do you think their role will be in this story?
> Where and when does the story take place?
> What is the basic plot (problem or goal?)

Students are then asked to stop periodically during their reading, perhaps at the end of each chapter, to check their "file" for needed revisions. It is important to go through this process with students as they are reading a novel, that is, to require that they record the page where their tentative file was formed and that they identify specific pages where new information required that they change or add to their file. This file should be discussed as a working guide to direct the reader's attention and to facilitate comprehension. It has been effective to suggest to adolescents that if they don't first establish and open a mental file, there will be no place to put new information. It will simply bounce off their foreheads and be lost if they have no file opened.

Processing through Multiple Readings

Blachowisc (1994) discussed a multiple reading strategy, creative problem solving (Lundsteen, 1974), that asks students to read a passage quickly to find out about characters. Students then reread to determine the goal or problem and, finally, they reread to determine solutions. There is discussion at each stage and the method seems to provide a good "walk-through" or modeling of actively predicting and confirming during reading. The focus on one factor at a time creates "wheat" and is easier than looking for all the elements of a story at once. Multiple reading of short passages can also allow for attention first to gist ("Okay, what's the basic story here—the big picture?") and then to detail in subsequent readings ("Now, what exactly happened and how?").

The use of story frames or probable passages (Gould, 1991) discussed earlier (Chapter 7) provides other ways to help students predict and manage story elements along with asking them to mark specific passages with meaning connections to the readers' prior experience, world knowledge or other stories they have read (Harvey & Goudis, 2000). Discussions of inference clues are very important so students can hear others' tell how they comprehend as they read, that is, what words cause them to recall something that helped them make sense of what they were reading. Students can hear others in discussions use their prior knowledge, their good logical thinking and their memory for similar work by the same author.

After presenting these strategies and involving students in their use, it is still always important to check the students' understanding by having them explain in their own words what they are doing and why (what-so what), to have guided practice to ensure understanding, and assignments requiring independent application. We cannot assume that just telling or showing once will cause adolescents to really understand and utilize these language processing strategies because "wisdom cannot be told" (Gragg, 1940). This is particularly true with those who have had difficulty in learning. They need more examples and more rehearsal before really claiming these strategies as their own.

■□ READING AND WRITING PARAGRAPHS

Most of our language tests, to be practical, include sentence level measures with a few requiring short passages. Unfortunately adolescents rarely are asked to function at the sentence level in their classes. At the very least, they are expected to understand paragraphs, so this must be addressed.

Understanding the Function of a Paragraph

Adolescents need to understand the function of a paragraph as a "distinct section or subdivision of a chapter, letter, etc., usually dealing with a particular point..." (McKechnie, 1983, p. 1298), to know that the reason for creating each paragraph is to make a specific point about the topic which ties those paragraphs together. To effectively work on paragraphs we must ensure that students appreciate why paragraphs exist and how to understand the information within them.

Listening and watching teachers provide a running commentary or "think aloud" as they write can introduce adolescents to the rhythm of paragraphs. It allows them to notice when a point has been made and the author regroups for a transition to a new point. It seems advisable to talk about "indenting here to start a new idea or thought" rather than using the word "paragraph" at this stage in order not to evoke past misconceptions about paragraphs if there are any. The goal is to help students discover the concept before dealing with the name. In observing the creation and marking of paragraphs, adolescents can develop a feel for the process. Adolescents can see where the writer indicates a new paragraph with space or indentation and hear the logic accompanying these meaning shifts. Students with language learning problems may, of course, need many such opportunities to observe paragraph making to allow for rule deduction. I might add, here, as I do with my adolescent clients, that I would need many examples (*many*) for learning about art, music and sports because I do not naturally "see" the underlying rules that govern those disciplines. It is important for instructors to appreciate this reality—that all of us have areas where we need many and varied presentations or exposure to new ideas—so they do not communicate irritation at having to make this extra effort for students.

Checking Understanding of Paragraph Boundaries

As a follow-up to the modeling and immersion in paragraphing, students are given material that is not marked in any way for paragraph boundaries. They are then asked to work in pairs to find the places where spaces or indentations should occur. It students do not think of this on their own, instructors can suggest that one of the pair read aloud to help them know where to divide the passage. If students cannot find the boundaries even with reading aloud, the instructor can read it aloud, noting pauses and discuss the reasons for those pauses, that is, as indications of change in meaning. When students begin to correctly identify the places to indent, then it is appropriate to begin using the word "paragraph" to name the concept that has been developed.

We have used a similar strategy for causing students to discover the importance of punctuation and spacing to mark word and sentence boundaries. Don Marquis wrote a column for the New York Evening Sun beginning in 1916 entitled, "archy and mehitabel" in which he used no capital letters because archy the cockroach in the newsroom there presumably wrote the column and could not manage the shift key on the typewriter. We have modeled our materials on his with the added stress of not providing spaces between words and ask students to read and discuss material so written.

(Example. "therearemanywaystoskinacatandIwilltellyouoneway.")

Eliciting Sentences and Expanding to Paragraphs on a Topic

One can also introduce paragraphs by first describing a real world scenario (Example: there was a recent civic project to build an aquarium), and then use probes to elicit various comments and/or main ideas which are expanded into paragraphs (see Box 8–2) of different types about the topic at hand, in this case, a new aquarium. For instance, one probe in this example takes the form of the following question: "Why did the city planners decide to build an aquarium?" Students are each asked to write a short reply and these are read aloud. The instructor selects one statement ("The city wanted to attract more tourists") to expand into a cause–effect paragraph that is written on chart paper and displayed on the wall. Other paragraph types are elicited, written and displayed around the room.

BOX 8–2: *Probes to Elicit Paragraph Types*

1. Why did the city planners want to build an aquarium? (Cause–effect)
2. What do you think they had to do in order to get this aquarium built? (Sequence)
3. Write about the difficulty of building on the riverbank. (Problem–solution)
4. What things do you think they wanted to include in the aquarium? (List/enumeration)
5. How would they want the aquarium to look and feel to people visiting? (Description)
6. Tell about how the city was before and after the aquarium. (Compare/contrast)

Matching Paragraphs Types with Different Topics

Students are given a second set of paragraphs written about a different topic (A flood). They are asked to read the second set of paragraphs and to match them to the original aquarium paragraphs on the wall. They then explain how the matching paragraphs are alike in spite of their different topics, what the purpose of each paragraph seems to be and how they know this is the purpose. ("In both paragraphs the authors were telling us what something looks like.")

Teaching Paragraph Types

Having elicited the students' own sentences about a topic, expanded those sentences into paragraphs, and further directed their attention to the various purposes of paragraphs through the matching exercises, the instructor introduces and directly teaches the paragraph types. The name of each paragraph type is given and attention is directed to specific words which signal each paragraph type. For instance, descriptive words are identified for descriptive paragraphs; words such as "because" and "so" signal cause/effect paragraphs; "first ... then ... after that" indicate a sequence; " ... several ways ... " indicate a list; "this ... that ... bigger than ... before—now" suggest comparison; and problem solution is often signaled by "so they ... ". There is discussion of the possible difficulties in distinguishing Cause/Effect paragraphs from Problem/Solution or List paragraphs from Sequence to direct students to the distinctive differences in these similar types. (Sequence paragraphs have to be in order—lists can be rearranged; problem–solution paragraphs have to have a problem and solution; cause and effect do not have a solution). Students are also challenged to use just the topic sentence in each paragraph to see if they can detect type, then to read the paragraph to confirm their initial impression.

Matching Again

The next step in this paragraph learning process asks students to match a set of paragraphs about a third topic (A Vacation) to the original paragraphs displayed. Although they have already matched paragraphs, it is important to reinforce that experience and the direct teaching with further practice. Again, the students match paragraphs and discuss how they identified the paragraphs, how they are alike, signal words and purposes.

Writing Paragraphs from Probes

Finally, students are assigned a topic, given probes and asked to write one example of each six paragraph types (see Box 8–3). Their paragraphs are read aloud, matched to the example paragraphs and named by type by other students.

This unit on paragraphs has proved effective in showing students that they already are expressing the intentions and purposes of various

---

BOX 8–3: *Probes for Writing Paragraphs About Baseball*

1. Tell what usually happens in baseball game from the beginning to the end. (Sequence)
2. List the major league ball parks. (List)
3. Describe one of the new ball parks. (Describe)
4. Compare Babe Ruth with Pete Rose. (Compare)
5. Talk about ball players high salaries and the effect on tickets. (Cause/Effect)
6. Discuss the high price of tickets and tell what can be done. (Problem/Solution)

paragraph types in their natural communication and they only have to learn to label them and to produce them consciously.

Collecting, Sorting and Analyzing Paragraphs

Follow-up lessons have included asking students to collect various paragraph types from their reading and writing to be used for sorting by type to support their understanding. Students have been asked to analyze paragraphs in worksheets requiring that they name the topic of the paragraph first, then identify the paragraph type and state the "point" that is being made about the topic in each paragraph, followed by telling the purpose of the author in writing this paragraph. This should be repeated with many paragraphs and students encouraged to discuss aspects of different types present in one paragraph. For instance, a cause/effect paragraph can also include lists of effects. A problem/solution may include comparisons of various solutions before deciding upon one.

Identifying Cohesion in Paragraphs

After students are able to identify the topic, the main idea or point which defines the paragraph, and to state the purpose of their own paragraphs and those they read in school materials, it seems appropriate to focus attention on cohesion. Students need to note specific signals that direct readers to tie information across sentence and/or thought boundaries. It is easy to find times within regular classroom routines for focusing students' attention to cohesion and, thus, to facilitate their active processing in reading. For instance, teachers can copy chapter summaries onto overhead transparencies and read them aloud as students listen and read along. Teachers can pause at "stopping places" and ask students to provide referents (for personal pronouns or for "pointing" words like "this ... these ... that one ... the ... "; for word omissions, etc.) to make the ties. Teachers can challenge students to find a specific number of "stopping places" as they listen to a passage, then to tie back (or forward) to referents. This effort can be made when introducing or reviewing a chapter which reinforces understanding of that content along with providing conscious practice in language processing. When students begin to consistently name referents in response to questions ("Him?"), then the concept of cohesion can be explained. It is helpful to talk about the purpose of adhesives and to equate their sticking "things" together to our tying words and their referents together. In addition, the concept of being coherent is discussed ("When someone is babbling, they are incoherent—we don't understand them."). These two concepts, being coherent and adhesives, explain cohesive ties. We make reading coherent by sticking word meanings together.

■□ READING AND WRITING COMPLEX STATEMENTS

The college student, Staci, described in Chapter 4 had particular difficulty understanding complex sentences in her textbooks. She could read the words fluently but often had no idea what was being said. Although more global strategies were helpful, such as previewing chapters and working actively on paragraphs Staci needed direct work on comprehending complex sentences.

For Staci's benefit and those of students having similar problems, complex sentences from expository texts can be displayed on overhead transparencies and read aloud. Summary statements from the end of textbook chapters or those of teachers' own creation for introducing (warming up) or reviewing a chapter or unit of study can be used for two purposes: learning how to process complex sentences and learning the pertinent concepts (wheat) important in the course of study.

Decombining Complex Sentences

The teacher, in this exercise, simply displays a sentence (*The effects of the damage from Sherman's march through Georgia have been etched in the minds of Southerners so much so that relations between them and those from Northern States ...*), reads it aloud and asks students first to tell the topic: "What is this sentence about—in one or two words?" (*Sherman's March*) and then asks the students to restate the sentence in one thought units: Tell me one thing you learned about the topic—just from reading this sentence." (*Sherman marched through Georgia ...*) Each one thought sentence is written below the source sentence on the overhead transparency. The students continue to "decombine" the sentence in this way by restating the complex sentence in single thought sentences: "Now someone give me another thought ... another ... " (*The effects of that march have been etched in the minds of Southerners. The effects are reflected still in relations between Southerners and Northerners).* Each sentence is written by the teacher so students can appreciate how to retrieve understandable concepts from the long, complex textbook sentences through this decombining (see Box 8–4). They will come to appreciate that, no matter how long and complex the sentence, there are individual, understandable thoughts that can be found.

Reconstructing Original Sentences and Discovering Connectors

After all single thoughts have been elicited and written, the teacher covers the original sentence and asks students to reconstruct it from their one thought sentences. ("Now, use these one thought sentences and try to recall the original sentence.") Students then compare their

---

BOX 8–4: *Sentence Decombining and Reconstructing*

"Like a dugout, a sod home or soddy, was warm in winter, cool in summer and was an island of color when wildflowers bloomed on its roof."

(Danzer et al., 1998, p. 398)

What is the topic?
　　A sod home

Tell me one thing you learn about a sod home from this sentence:
　　It was like a dugout.
　　It was also called a "soddy."
　　It was warm in winter.
　　It was cool in summer
　　Wildflowers bloomed on its roof.
　　It was an island of color.

Now use these sentences to reconstruct the original sentence.

---

reconstructed sentences to the original, which is uncovered and shown on the overhead again (see Box 8–4). The attempt to reconstruct the original sentence directs attention to the words connecting the individual thoughts (so much so that ...). Students discover that they can reproduce the same individual thoughts but change the relationships at times, if they change the connector words in their recall. This is another appropriate place to directly teach and discuss various cohesive ties and their impact on meaning. The difference between tying thoughts together with "and" versus "but" provokes good appreciation of the function of these words for instance.

In Staci's case, the sentence decombining and reconstruction seemed to direct attention to both the individual thoughts and their connectors. It was interesting that after engaging in these exercises, Staci's oral reading changed. At the beginning of our work she had read a passage from a respiratory therapy class textbook and she read so quickly that she did not seem to be actively processing the material. After engaging in sentence combining for several weeks, however, Staci read from the same book but with pauses reflecting attention to individual thoughts within sentences. She had begun to decombine the complex sentences as she read which was especially interesting because we had never discussed her inappropriate reading rate and phrasing.

Decombining Main Idea Statements

Expository chapters often provide the "main idea" at the beginning of a chapter to direct students attention to the "wheat" before they read.

Those are important sentences to read closely to provide good reasons for sentence decombining. It is important, in this exercise, to discourage paraphrasing in favor of restating facts in a way that is faithful to the original sentence (see Box 8–5). Many students offer information they already know about a topic and need to practice confining themselves to what they learn from reading the sentence. This is a good discipline for those students who bring rich experience and information to school enabling them in the early years of school to answer many questions without reading the text.

BOX 8–5: *Main Ideas Decombined*

1. The government looks after the interests of the people.
   (a) The topic is government
   (b) We learn from this sentence that government looks after the interests of the people.
2. In a monarchy, the people are ruled by a person who has inherited his or her power.
   (a) The topic is a monarchy.
   (b) These are the facts we learn from this sentence about a monarchy:
       People in a monarchy are ruled by a person.
       That ruler has inherited his or her power.
           (O'Connor & Goldberg, 1980, p. 14).
3. Two processes that help narrow down inputs are selective attention and feature extraction.
   (a) The topic is two processes.
   (b) These are the facts that we learn about the two processes:
       The processes are called selective attention and feature extraction.
       These processes help narrow down inputs.
4. Decay is the fading away of a memory and, if it occurs at all, is not the main reason for forgetting.
   (a) The topic is decay.
   (b) The facts are as follows:
       Decay is the fading away of a memory.
       Decay may not occur.
       Decay is not the main reason for forgetting.
           (Perrin, L. [Ed.], 1986, p. 75)

(continued)

BOX 8–5: *(continued)*

5. The Grand Canyon was formed by miners in search of valuable minerals.
   (a) The topic is the Grand Canyon.
   (b) The facts are as follows:
   The Grand Canyon was formed by miners.
   These miners were searching for valuable minerals.
6. Distance from the equator, altitude, and distance from the ocean all affect the climate of a place.
   (a) The topic is climate of a place.
   (b) The facts are as follows:
   Distance from the equator affects the climate of a place.
   Distance from the ocean affects the climate of a place.
   Altitude affects the climate of a place.
   (Banks et al., 1995, p. 40)

Decombining Conversational Questions

Question decombining can be introduced by using spontaneous student generated questions that allow learning of the new strategy within familiar information and language.

"What are we having for lunch?"

(a) The topic is lunch;
(b) The fact is we are having something for lunch;
(c) The direction tells us we have to tell what we are having for lunch.

After discovering the two major parts of statements, and adding the direction to make the three parts of conversational questions, it is easier for students to apply the decombining strategy with more difficult text questions. In any case, students need practice, especially those with language difficulty, to increase awareness of the three important parts of a question: topic, facts, and directions.

■□ UNDERSTANDING AND ANSWERING REVIEW QUESTIONS

Review questions typically provided after sections and at the end of chapters in social studies and science texts can be analyzed in much the same way as complex sentences. The student is asked 1) to identify the topic ("Just one or two words, please. What is this question about? What is the topic?") and then 2) to tell the facts ("What do we know about this topic—just from reading this question?"). Students need to confine their facts to those inherent in the question just as they do in explaining facts in main idea statements referred to above. Finally, in decombining questions (see Box 8–6), they are asked 3) to explain the implicit direction in the question ("Tell what we must do to answer the question").

One student's social studies text provided on the first page of every chapter, the main idea and two questions to direct students to "wheat" as they read. It was easy and productive to practice decombining of statements and questions presented as a regular introduction to each new chapter. The student knew to always identify the topic and the given facts and, in questions, to also attend to the direction word or words that told her to do something. This provided language practice within the usual routine of reading a new chapter.

BOX 8–6: *Question Decombining with Text Questions*

Question: Why is Lincoln considered the "Great Emancipator." when he was not an antislavery sympathizer at the beginning of his career and his wife's family owned slaves?

Topic:	Lincoln
Facts:	Lincoln is considered the "Great Emancipator."
	Lincoln did not sympathize with the antislavery movement early in his career.
	Lincoln's wife's family owned slaves.
Direction:	I must explain why Lincoln is considered the "Great Emancipator" in spite of his early political sympathies and his wife's family's slaveowning.

Creating Right Questions for Wrong Answers

Close, accurate reading of questions ensures that students are better able to show their knowledge and are not penalized for misunderstanding the language in questions. Students are asked, in a further effort to enhance their awareness of the information in questions, to note their wrong answers on tests and to create a question that goes with their answer. This exercise directs their attention to what they noticed and what they missed in their reading of the original question (see Box 8–7). For instance, students sometimes misread the direction word (what ...) and provide an answer appropriate to a different direction word (when). As they try to create a question to match their wrong answer they must notice the direction word. Another way students can go wrong in answering is to quickly identify the topic of the question and leap to a point that was emphasized about that topic in class discussion. Perhaps because of anxiety in test taking, they don't even notice that this question does not include that expected fact. For instance, the discussion in class may have stressed that Lincoln had extreme difficulty with McClellan, a general who could not be shaken out of his inaction and would not move his troops as commanded. So, in answer to the question, "Who was the last general hired by the North in the Civil War?" this student might attend to the words "Civil War" and "general" then leap to the conclusion that this is the expected question requiring an explanation about why Lincoln was dissatisfied with General McClellan. In that case, the student's mistake would result from neglecting the fact in the question.

BOX 8–7: *Wrong Answers Exercise*

Read the following questions and wrong answers. Write the question that better matches this answer.

Original Question:	What general caused Lincoln difficulty in the Civil War?
Wrong Answer:	President Lincoln was frustrated by his unwillingness or inability to take needed action.
Matching Question:	The student assumed that this was the question: *Why was Lincoln so upset with General McClellan?*

Discovering Direction Words and Writing Answers

Teaching students to understand questions is important to ensure that they understand what is being asked. Understanding the question, however, does not always ensure that students will produce good answers. Tattershall & Prendeville (1993) reported that a middle school student learned to consistently decombine questions into their three constituent parts but could not supply an appropriate answer even when she knew the content. This student could identify the word "compare" as the direction word in questions, but she didn't know how to write a good response to the direction to "compare" two ideas. This student had learned to say what she needed to say in decombining questions, but she really didn't know what these words meant in order to respond with an appropriate answer.

Prendeville devised a plan for collecting and studying, with her student, the review questions in her social studies textbook. They grouped the questions by direction words with similar intent ("Tell ... explain ... list ... describe"). Prendeville modeled good answers for the various direction words and then, with her student, identified the critical features of these good answers. She taught, for example, that before one can compare two ideas, people or terms, one has to introduce and describe each idea, person or term. Strichart and Mangrum II (1993), in a similar effort, directed students' attention to direction words and made suggestions for helping students to appreciate those words requiring the same type of response (discuss, describe, tell ...) as contrasted with those that are similar but require slightly different responses (summarize, list, outline) (see Box 8–8).

BOX 8–8: *Noticing Direction Words and Writing Good Answers*

(after Strichart & Mangrum II, 1993, pp. 324–326)

DIRECTION WORDS	ANSWERS
discuss, describe, explain, tell	write as much as you know
summarize	a short statement with important ideas
list	simply list what is asked for
outline	give the main points and supporting facts in outline form
diagram and illustrate	make a drawing and label the parts
	illustrate with a drawing and/or give an example to show the meaning
trace	state how things happened in order
compare, relate	tell how things are alike, how they are connected
contrast	tell how things are different
criticize, evaluate, justify	write about the value of something
criticize & evaluate	tell the positive and negative
justify	provide reasons to explain

Discovering Patterns to Guide Answering

Prendeville (Tattershall & Prendeville, 1993) reported that she and her student learned, in collecting and classifying text questions by direction word, that the authors of the student's textbook favored a small, finite group of question types. This discovery simplified the teaching and learning of appropriate answers and the student began to produce appropriate answers to this closed set of questions. She also, presumably, learned something about discovering patterns in a textbook to guide her studying.

Modeling and Analyzing Good Answers

Another approach for helping students learn to write more effective answers asks teachers to collect answers to be displayed and discussed. The time spent in discussing answers for their effectiveness and discovering the shared characteristics of "good" answers is more helpful than teachers simply presenting guidelines to be followed. A student with language learning problems is certainly better served by presentation of many examples and discussion leading to a list of requirements to guide the answering of questions in that class. Teachers may discover through this process that many students profit from time spent on formulating answers. Students who know how to accurately read a question and how to produce good answers that meet the criteria discussed in their class are able to focus on curricular content without the interference of language processing problems.

■☐ WORD AND SYLLABLE PROCESSING

Many adolescents have insufficient vocabulary knowledge which contributes to comprehension problems in reading and listening. When inadequate word knowledge makes reading unsatisfying these students avoid reading, which of course, sets up a negative spiral. Not reading limits their exposure and opportunity to learn new words which then interferes with subsequent reading attempts and so on. Some of these students have strengths in word decoding or sight word memory and can read words that they do not understand. Because they can read even unfamiliar words, they do not always identify those words they do not understand. They don't identify the problem and then don't look for context clues or look up the word.

One young man recovering from a head trauma read a passage fluently and accurately. When asked if there were any new or hard words in the passage, he said "No." When asked to explain the meaning of specific words selected from the reading, however, it was clear that he did not know their meaning. His approach to reading suggested a view of reading as an oral performance rather than a meaning–making process. Bert who had significant learning problems in math and also attention problems (see Chapter 4) showed this same pattern of reading or listening without monitoring for unknown vocabulary. Both young men seemed fooled by their ability to pronounce the words accurately as they read. They seemed to have a strength in decoding the surface of language and to feel that this was adequate.

Monitoring for Unknown Words

Students who do not monitor for unknown words need assignments that require their locating new vocabulary in reading or listening about familiar topics. Rather than engaging them weekly in learning twenty new words selected by someone else, they are better served to find their own needed word meanings. It may help to collaborate with these students to increase their vigilance for new words in class discussions and to find acceptable ways to ask about the meanings of those new words. An appropriate assignment is to ask these students to write new words from a discussion, check the dictionary and then confirm the meaning with the teacher.

A parent, an instructor who knows a student well, or a peer, can start the process of self-monitoring for new words by first identifying words the student probably does not know in a passage. The adult collaborator can then challenge the student to listen or read to find that specific number of new words. The teacher can check understanding of any targeted words the student did not identify as unfamiliar, and the student can keep a keep a running record of the percentage of new words he or she identified. A follow-up to modeling by the teacher is to ask the student to become the tutor and work with a younger peer. The student/tutor first reads a passage and predicts which words the peer/tutee may not understand, then asks the "tutee" to listen or read and try to identify a specific number of new words.

These monitoring activities focus on the first part of the problem solving process—identifying the problem, the words the student may be able to read but not understand. We hope the focus on understanding rather than just pronouncing words may also change the student's view of reading. Practically, if we do not help students identify independently what they know and do not know about words they read or hear, they may not develop effective vocabulary learning strategies.

Reading the Context for Word Meaning

Students who improve their monitoring for unknown words, can then work at learning new vocabulary along with those who have insufficient vocabulary and naturally identify unknown words. Both groups can practice using context—reading around the words to develop a prediction about what the word might mean. Nippold (1988) suggested that words are learned by direct teaching or through contextual abstraction, a process in which a word is heard or read repeatedly and the context is used for inferring meaning. This repeated reading for contextual abstraction could serve as a "warm-up" for looking for the word in a thesaurus or dictionary. Having some idea about its meaning in context allows students to better select the pertinent definition. This is an important step for many who have been told to simply "Look it up." For those with limited vocabulary and other language weaknesses the dictionary can be imposing and frustrating. If they are guided in the process of predicting word meanings from the context, learning to use guide words to find the correct page quickly, and then searching the multiple meanings with their predictions in mind, they can use the dictionary more effectively.

Appreciating Word Usage in Sentences

Students with limited academic language skills can find the word in the dictionary but not identify the correct definition, find the correct definition but not understand its meaning, and/or can find the correct definition and understand the meaning but not be able to correctly use the word in a sentence. One such student demonstrated the limited value of learning words by definition only when she responded to a suggestion with this remark, "I'm cognizant, I'm cognizant." She knew something about the meaning of the word "cognizant" but was unsure about how to use it. Students need to hear words used in a variety of sentences and contexts before they can really appreciate the word's meaning and be confident in producing their own appropriate comments with that word. A definition and one example sentence is insufficient. Instructors need to understand that the definition does not always lead to appropriate usage, that contextual abstraction may require more context than is usually given, and that combining use of context, definitions and many examples of the word in sentences is most effective for vocabulary learning and essential for those without a natural talent for vocabulary development, that is, those who need to be taught.

Learning New Vocabulary in a Top-Down Sequence

In a class for college bound students with known learning problems, a colleague and I used the following sequence for teaching new vocabulary (see Box 8–9). From a list of probable topics of discussion among college students, we selected one and I wrote a passage on the topic. As I wrote, I included vocabulary that was appropriate to the topic but might be new for this group. I read my passage aloud as the students read along using their own copies. We discussed the passage first to establish a general context for the new vocabulary, then I read each new word aloud and asked if someone could use the word in a sentence. The other instructor and I then provided several more example sentences for each new word. The students were given a list of the words and, in pairs, took turns using the words in sentences within a timed exercise. The students listed, after this timed sentence making exercise, the words they felt they now knew well enough to understand in a passage or to use in a sentence of their own making. The remaining words that many students seemed confident about were written on the board. Students who could and the two instructors created more sentences with these words. In the next class this same sequence was repeated but, this time, my colleague had written a different paragraph on the same topic to provide another meaning context for the same words. The students had more success in providing individual sentences in the group and then using the words in their own sentences in pairs. On this second class meeting, the students again identified the words that they seemed confident about using in sentences and those that they still found difficult. They then looked up the words in a thesaurus first and then in a dictionary. They finished by working in pairs to create two sentences for each word.

This experience in learning ten new words required work for these young adults and showed the difficulty that must be presented in the often used weekly assignment for middle school students to learn 20 new vocabulary words. With very little contextual support to make the words meaningful, they typically must learn those words by using definitions and selecting words for cloze sentences. Even in our sequence with more ways to learn the word and more active rehearsal, our college bound students with learning problems could have used several more lessons on their ten new words to really master them. Our lesson sequence did seem to offer a realistic approach to teaching vocabulary. A variation on this sequence asks students to bring in their own passages with new words marked, discussing that passage and working on sentences, then writing a second paragraph using the student–identified words for the second session.

BOX 8–9: *A Top–Down Vocabulary Lesson Sequence*

1. Select an appropriate topic and write a paragraph.
2. Underline probable new vocabulary.
3. Read the paragraph aloud to present words in context.
4. Ask students to use the words in sentences.
5. Instructor provides more sentences for each word.
6. Ask students to work in pairs to use the words in sentences.
7. Repeat the process with a different paragraph and same new vocabulary.
8. Repeat the process with students providing passages and words.

Understanding Principles for Teaching New Vocabulary

Wallace (1982) discusses several principles for teaching new vocabulary in a second language which seem applicable to learning vocabulary in a first language (see Box 8–10). 1) The teacher must be clear about the aim of a vocabulary learning lesson. Is the student supposed to simply recognize the word, be able to recall it, pronounce it, spell it, relate it to an object or concept, use it in sentences at an appropriate level of formality, be aware of its connotations? With the often used vocabulary learning lesson of twenty words unrelated to one topic and presented out of context one wonders about the goal. 2) The teacher has to decide on the number of new words to teach. Wallace (1982) notes that the frustration level in reading is evoked when ten percent of the words are unknown; therefore, it is important to limit the number of new words. 3) The teacher should consider vocabulary that is needed by students, its frequency of occurrence, availability and learnability. If a word is obscure and seldom encountered, the student may not have the opportunity to use it and learn it well. If the teacher wants to fill the student's head with exotic words to bring him "above the crowd," then it is the responsibility of the teacher to make those words available through frequent use and exposure within a supportive context with enough opportunity for learning to occur. 4) Another principle in teaching vocabulary, according to Wallace (1982) is that words must be presented so that the meaning is clear and unambiguous, which again requires supplying sufficient, meaningful context or situation. 5) A fifth principle in word learning is that we usually learn words "approximately" at first and gradually increase our precision in using and understanding a word. The ZPD, zone of proximal development, (Vygotsky, 1978; Wells, 1999) seems clearly appropriate as does the old–new balance in suggesting that new words be added within the context of known topics when possible and with extensive opportunities for the learner to appreciate and incorporate words into existing lexicons. Wallace suggests that words always be taught within a lesson rather than aside from the lesson and that teachers select words that are well supported and critical to the meaning. He also suggests that

---

BOX 8–10: *Guidelines for Teaching New Vocabulary*

(Adapted from Wallace, 1982)

1. Be clear about the goal: recognition, recall, use in sentence, define ...?
2. Limit the number of new words.
3. Choose appropriate vocabulary (practical, opportunities to use, learnable).
4. Supply unambiguous, clear context for words.
5. Expect approximate understanding and work for refinement.
6. Teach words within a lesson on one topic.
7. Include new vocabulary selected by students.

students self-select other unknown words at the end of the lesson, after overall meaning and teacher selected words have been addressed.

There appear to be two levels for learning new vocabulary. Working on a functional, practical level we should encourage and reinforce students in identifying their own needed new vocabulary. Until students are consistently identifying their own problem words, vocabulary learning will not be functional for them. In addition to encouraging monitoring for words within known topics and familiar experiences, instructors can expose students to more exotic vocabulary. This is a more academic level of vocabulary learning. Several cautions should be kept in mind, however. Students should notice when they don't know a word, wherever they encounter it. This is basic. No matter how many exotic words they can match to definitions and learn out of context, these words will probably not be used if students aren't monitoring for word meaning in their reading and listening. The second suggestion is to aim for real understanding of words acquired with many presentations and supportive contexts at the discourse and sentence levels rather than simply focusing on quantity of new words. And finally, students and instructors need to clearly understand that knowing the dictionary meaning, however helpful that can be, often does not teach one how to use the word appropriately. We all need to be cognizant of the need for learning word usage by reading and hearing the word many times within a variety of contexts.

Focusing on Words with Limited Awareness of Syllable and Sound

Many adolescents persist in having difficulty reading words accurately and seem particularly wary of long words. They seem to look at the whole word in their reading and to neglect fine distinctions at the syllable and sound level. They often "telescope" words by omitting the middle syllable ("contrate" for concentrate) do not notice consonant clusters ("bought" vs. "brought"), or neglect word endings. It is interesting that these students sometimes show this same neglect in their oral pronunciation of words and seem to slur parts of some words as they talk (bro*ther*, ano*ther*). Interestingly these students improve their speech clarity when asked to repeat phrases with these previously slurred words. It is as if they can produce these sounds in words but do not actively monitor at this level of language unless called upon to make themselves clear. Then they focus on the sounds in syllables. Sometimes students produce a word in their oral reading that is visually similar to the text word and makes sense in the sentence so they do not notice the mistake ("He was talking himself through it" may be replaced with "He was taking himself through it.").

There are a variety of suggestions as to why these kinds of mistakes are made. Clearly there is limited phonologic awareness which some may call an auditory processing problem. This behavior seems to fit both descriptions but neither seems to explain why some people do not seem to notice the syllable and sound level of words. My observations of many adolescents and adults suggest that many of these kinds of speakers and readers are practical learners who are meaning makers and good nonverbal problem solvers. They seem to have an attention style reflected by their focus on content and meaning and they are satisfied with their search for meaning down to and including words. They have difficulty, however, noticing the less meaningful smaller segments of language: syllables and sounds. "What is 'eck?' " they might wonder when asked to focus on a rime pattern, a language segment that is smaller than a word and is part of a system based on sound but not on meaning. I view these kinds of learners as "whole worders" who are good thinkers but have limited patience with nonsense. Work directed to sound patterns that are not based on meaning may seem like nonsense to those with this attention style. Directing their attention to the syllable and sound level of language is important for refining oral pronunciation, and for reading and spelling. Otherwise, because of their attention style, the "whole worders" among us would never notice distinctions in similar words.

Directing Attention to Syllable and Sound Through Word Comparisons

Word comparison, modified from one suggested by Bettelheim and Zelan (1982), is a helpful technique for the "whole worder" group. When a student misread a word in oral reading, Bettelheim would ask why he or she had produced a particular word instead of reading the actual word in the text. The question seemed to suggest that the misreading had been purposeful, signaling some personal motive in Bettelheim's description. I am not convinced that there is an underlying motive for the misreading, but the question posed by Bettelheim caused students to look again, more closely, at the actual text word and, sometimes, to self-correct their reading miscue.

Causing students to compare their miscues with the author's intended word is tailored to that reader's mistake and offers personalized, relevant practice in noticing critical differences between words. Miscues often reflect a reader's neglect of fine distinctions between visually similar words, so placing the words side by side for comparison directs attention to these syllable and sound level differences. With this opportunity to compare words, students sometimes notice the critical difference between their miscue and the text word and self-correct on their second guess. In these cases, the word comparison technique seems to train students' attention more than to teach them how to read the word. Whole worders may be able to read words, then, but not to notice distinctions between similar words unless placed in this problem solving situation.

The student with serious phonologic awareness problems may not self-correct so easily but will profit from these opportunities to discover differences and shared patterns in words—characteristics they may never notice on their own because of their focus on whole words. They begin to hone their attention to the exact part of words that is causing them difficulty and be ready to learn that vowel pattern, consonant cluster or suffix that was previously unnoticed.

After students are given an opportunity to self-correct by simply comparing their miscue (read aloud to them and written next to the target text word), they make a second guess that is also written for use in comparison and finally, they are given a clue word that shares a pattern with and can be used to read the text word. Sometimes students's guesses at this point are very close but they are accenting the wrong syllable. If given a sentence with the word, they can recognize a word that is in their working vocabulary.

Word comparison highlights what needs to be noticed at the syllable/sound levels of words (see Boxes 8–11 and 8–12). It is good attention practice but, by itself, does not teach the words. Once the students notice and can correct miscues through word comparison, they may need extensive guided practice in searching and collecting other words with shared intraword patterns. They need to read and sort words into

---

BOX 8–11: *Word Comparison*

HOW:

- Do a word comparison exercise with the hard words that occurred in an oral reading or compare the student's miscues (guesses during reading) with the actual words in the book.
- Write the first hard word (the actual word from the reading). ("wreak")
- Write the students miscue ("first guess") next to the actual word.
- Read the miscue aloud (This was your first guess "week").
- Then ask for a second guess.
- ("Now look at the actual word and make a second guess.")
- Write the second guess ("wreak") and read this second guess aloud for the student.
- If needed, write a clue word with the necessary shared pattern ("Use this word, 'deck' to guess the word.").
- If needed, make a sentence with the word to allow use of context.
- Show on the Word Comparison Sheet when the student read the word. (second guess?, clue word?, sentence?)

(continued)

BOX 8–11: *(continued)*

EXAMPLE:
- Hard *actual* word: "Wreck"
- Guesses: "week" "wreek"
- Clue word: "deck"
- Sentence clue: "We had a terrible wreck in our car."

WHY:
- To direct attention to patterns within words.
- To show the shared patterns among words.
- To encourage using known words to unlock unknown words.
- To encourage use of sentence context.
- To direct attention to good reading attempts, that is, how close the student may be to the word even if not totally correct or which part he/she noticed in the actual word.
- To have a continuing record of the student's word reading.

BOX 8–12: *Word Comparison Sheets*

(Mark column where word is figured out.)
Name of student_____
Date started_____

Actual word:	First guess	Second Guess	Clue word	Sentence

WORD SORTING
HOW:
- Select a group of about 20 words from a word bank resulting from word comparisons, collected misspelled words from student writing or targeted vocabulary in various subjects.
- Write the words on cards for sorting.

(continued)

- Select several words that can be grouped (rhyming words, same first letter, same vowel sound and spelling, same vowel sound but different spelling, same number of letters, similar meaning, part of speech, etc.) and place them in the same area on a table.
- Read your group of words aloud and ask the student to try to find or provide another word that fits in your group. If the student selects a word that does not fit your intended category, keep providing other words that fit until the student consistently selects or suggests appropriate words for the group.
- Ask the student to explain how the words go together, that is, why they are grouped together. If the student suggests a different category but all words fit, celebrate! Tell them that they have noticed something about these words that you did not and that, because all the words fit with their classification, it works. Then tell them why you put these words together.
- Start a word group book or file. Name the groups and put all the words in that group. Later you can consult your book or file to see if any of the old words also fit into new groups that are identified later.

WHY:
- This activity directs attention to the shared characteristics of words. Rather than learning each word individually, an inefficient strategy given all the words one has to learn, students learn patterns or characteristics they may recognize in new words they read or spell.

various shared patterns, to spell those words with the shared patterns visible and then to spell and read the words without patterns available to check their having attended to and internalized the shared patterns.

After students have discovered and named the categories of words in discovered groups based on shared patterns, they can be challenged to order them from specific to general or vice versa or to their degree of severity, intensity, size, and so forth in order to increase awareness of nuance and subtlety (Gould, 1991; Englert & Raphael, 1988; Klein, 1985; Johnson & Pearson, 1984).

■❏ WORKING ON SPELLING

There are many students with language based learning difficulties that include problems in spelling. There are other students whose language learning seems to be obvious only in spelling. Parents who complain that school reform has ruined spelling and that teachers should return to the "good old fashioned ways" feel that new approaches are the problem. It is interesting to ask these parents if they know anyone their age or older who is a bad speller. They have to agree that many of us who went through the traditional spelling programs did not learn to be good spellers. In these parents' defense, many students whose spelling words are chosen from their own writing or who are required to learn and proofread their writing for a core of high frequency words identified by grade level or other functional approaches, are also not learning to spell. Spelling skill seems to separate those who come into the world either wired for spelling or not. There seem to be many people who have language learning problems at this level of language. Those who have a natural propensity for noticing patterns for spelling do well with any method that provides a minimal number of examples. With this exposure, they simply learn to spell. They may not be able to explicitly explain the rules that guide their spelling, except for "I before E except after C," which seems to be the one most people can recite on request, but they "just know" when to double consonants or to mark long A with ai (rain) or ay (way) or eigh (weight) without being able to explain how they do it. There probably are the "haves" and the "have nots" when it comes to spelling. Those who did not receive the talent for spelling at birth need to be taught. If they are adolescents they may need continued teaching and/or accommodations that will keep them in the "spelling club," a refinement of Frank Smith's "Literacy Club."

Preparing for Using Spell Checkers

A practical goal for many adolescents and adults with weak spelling skills is to work toward producing misspellings that approximate the word closely enough to allow use of spell checkers. Free writing exercises (Elbow, 1973), followed by students' proofing for spelling can reveal the type and percentage of misspellings they identify. Students need to know which words are misspelled in order to use hand held spell checkers when computers are not available. Helping students study and discover their misspelling types in order to increase their proofing accuracy can enable them to independently use the aids available. Checking their writing samples for the percentage of misspellings that may be identified allows for correct word choices by a spell checker and is important. Many weak spellers need extensive help before they can effectively use a spell checker. A caution here: some spellers spell words as they sound. Their spellings look and sound like the intended word, so they may not identify them. They have to know that hand held spell checkers, that depend on the student's identifying and typing in the needed word, may not work as well as spell checkers within word processing programs that identify the misspellings for you.

Working Directly to Improve Spelling

Adolescents and adults who want to improve spelling need to appreciate first that patience and motivation are required. Language learning problems at the syllable and sound level of language are not easily ameliorated. It can be done but weak spellers need *many* opportunities to discover patterns, to collect many words sharing those patterns to enhance attention to this level of language, and many opportunities to actively sort words into patterns, to spell by pattern and to spell self-correct and write the words highlighting the pattern they need to learn. It is a formidable project and requires clear and serious motivation. The collaborating partner should discuss the efficacy of working toward using spell checkers as described above as a first goal, with students deciding after reaching that goal if they want to work for independent spelling ability beyond that. For the brave and committed this work can be interesting and challenging. New insights intended for spelling improvement also support more precise pronunciation of multisyllabic words and improve word awareness for reading.

Attending to Syllables to Guide Spelling

Those with weak spelling invariably depend on whole word visual memory to guide their spelling. They wince visibly when presented with a "long" word and try to reproduce it as a whole. When the instructor models identifying syllables ("Notice and feel your chin drop for each syllable in the word "Sep tem ber"), even those with severe reading and spelling problems show ability to correctly identify the number of syllables in a word. They seem to have the sense of syllable, even when they are not sure of that term, but they often do not try to spell words in a syllable by syllable fashion. This kind of speller often frowns when they read a word they have written signaling dissatisfaction with the spelling. When asked which part of the word seems wrong to them, they will often gesture nonspecifically ("Somewhere around here.") suggesting that they have a memory for the whole word but are unsure of the exact letters or sounds within it. The first important step in spelling more efficiently then, is to help these students focus on syllables within words. I often suggest to them that they must "take a small bite" in order not to "choke on the whole word." The students are guided in identifying words with one, two, three and four syllables. I prefer using "chin drops" to note syllables but many adolescents and adults seem to prefer clapping for each syllable or tapping their finger on their arm to show each syllable. Obviously, it is unimportant which method is used just so students become proficient in identifying the syllables. Then they must learn to say each syllable to guide their spelling of that part of the word and to consistently spell by syllables. A benchmark for many students is becoming consistent in spelling syllables phonetically showing their use of syllable and sound to guide their spelling. Their visual memory then can supplement their use of sound to self-correct their spellings. Even natural spellers use their whole word memory to identify and correct misspellings. However, many adolescents need to learn to utilize the auditory sense of sound at the syllable level before depending on visual memory.

Vertical spelling exercises are effective in focusing on spelling by syllable (see Box 8–13). Students are engaged, in this approach, in identifying the number of syllables shown by lines written in a vertical array. Students then say the first syllable aloud and spell that syllable on the first line. They then say the second syllable aloud and spell it on the second line (under the first). They continue this vertical spelling until the word is spelled. Students are then asked to read their spelling, syllable by syllable. Instructors must sometimes read their spellings for them. This step is critical for identifying misspellings and requires practice.

Students invariably remember the word that was intended but must learn to read exactly what they have written. Then they check their spelling by writing the correct word, in vertical fashion, next to their first attempt. Comparing misspellings with correct spelling, syllable by syllable, reveals the parts of the word that the student knows as well as the parts they need to learn. Rather than consider just right—wrong words, the student focuses on the patterns that need work and the patterns that are probably already known and are available for other spellings when needed. This comparison causes selective attention necessary for learning to spell. Students gain confidence in attempting longer words when they discover that words are made up of smaller, more manageable parts—syllables.

BOX 8–13: *Vertical Spelling Exercises*

1. Say the word and write lines to show syllables.
2. Arrange syllable lines in a vertical array (2nd syllable written under 1st, 3rd under 2nd ...)
3. Pronounce each syllable and spell/write it.
4. Then read the spelling—syllable by syllable.
5. Make a second guess based on the reading.
6. Check by writing correct spelling, vertically, beside first attempt.
7. Note the correct spelling and repeat steps 1–6.
8. Search for and collect words with shared syllables.

Writing to Spell

Weak spellers must be encouraged and supported in their writing attempts. We have required adults to keep journals and to write daily to make up for the limited writing they have done and to help them feel less anxious when writing. In many cases, the spelling is either emotionally charged for them or the effort of spelling makes writing difficult. We have suggested in some cases that they use newspaper headlines and simply write sentences using those words; that they read a short passage and write a summary consulting the passage for needed words. We have also guided invented spellings and celebrated good mistakes that show improvement in approximating the conventional spelling. Many adolescents and adults have developed skill in avoiding reading and writing and it is difficult to work around their resistance to showing their weakest area.

A spelling program was designed for a group of adolescents with this requirement. We wanted students whose listening comprehension was good but whose word decoding in reading and spelling was weak. This group included five adolescent boys who complained freely about the first requirement, to free write for increasingly longer periods starting with one minute intervals of writing without stopping. We explained that this was not a composition class and the writing did not have to make sense. They just had to write and keep writing during the timed periods ("We just want you to keep the words coming out of your head, down your arm and out your fingers!"). It was interesting that after a few weeks, I spoke to one of the boys about the writing acknowledging that I knew they had complained about it at first and he responded with a smile, "I didn't like it but you know what? I can write a whole page without stopping now." The fifteen minute time period became the standard that apparently evoked the longest piece of writing this young man had ever produced and he seemed happy with that accomplishment. We planned the free writing so the students would not inhibit use of words they could not spell. The requirement that they keep writing caused them to use many words from their known vocabulary but ones that they could not spell and had probably avoided in writing assignments.

The second step in this writing to spell program asked students to proofread their pieces for spelling and to circle the words they thought were misspelled. Then the instructors read their pieces and boxed the remaining misspelled words providing a running visible record of the proportion of their misspellings from their working vocabularies that the students could identify.

After the misspellings were identified by circling and boxing, the students were asked to make a second attempt at spelling each word. Then they were given the correct spelling so they could type each misspelling. Type one spellings were those that the students circled and could self-correct. These were considered words that they had learned but had not yet used enough to erase the old misspelling. Type two spellings were those that the students had circled but could not self-correct in their second attempt. They could get help for spelling these words because they knew they were misspelled and they seemed ready to learn them. Type three spellings were not identified by the students but the instructor had boxed them. Second attempts sometimes resulted in self-correction (a three plus) but the students did not seem to be as ready to learn them because they had not noticed them in their proofing. The traffic light analogy can be used here to show that these were not as yellow as number two spellings. Type four was added at the suggestion of a student who reminded us that a weak speller might circle a correct word.

Intervention for spelling was organized in this way. Type one (circled–corrected) and Type four (circled a correct spelling) were grouped. To ensure practice on this core set of words, students wrote sentences to dictation, proofed and self-corrected. They learned to spell type one words on their first try and to trust their correct spellings of type four. Types two and three were grouped and students were engaged in word sorting to discover and practice word patterns, in searching and collecting more words with the patterns, then learning and spelling words in pattern groups.

This writing to spell approach seemed practical in teaching adolescents to spell words within their working vocabularies (see Box

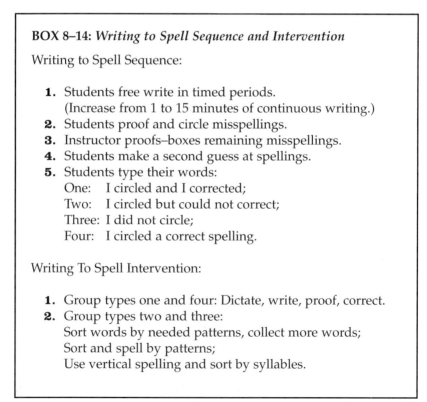

BOX 8–14: *Writing to Spell Sequence and Intervention*

Writing to Spell Sequence:

1. Students free write in timed periods.
   (Increase from 1 to 15 minutes of continuous writing.)
2. Students proof and circle misspellings.
3. Instructor proofs–boxes remaining misspellings.
4. Students make a second guess at spellings.
5. Students type their words:
   One: I circled and I corrected;
   Two: I circled but could not correct;
   Three: I did not circle;
   Four: I circled a correct spelling.

Writing To Spell Intervention:

1. Group types one and four: Dictate, write, proof, correct.
2. Group types two and three:
   Sort words by needed patterns, collect more words;
   Sort and spell by patterns;
   Use vertical spelling and sort by syllables.

8–14). One can add to the program by identifying and increasing the percentage of words amenable to using spell checkers; by expanding word use through dictation or writing summaries of reading or listening on known topics with new vocabulary; writing on new topics with old known vocabulary, and so on.

■□ SUMMARY

This chapter has emphasized the need for direct teaching and supervised practice of strategies for processing and producing academic language—skills that are necessary for adolescents' success for language demands that exceed those of short, casual interchanges in social conversation. Some students undoubtedly manage the linguistic leap to higher level language processing but, without teaching of strategies, many students cannot. These students need to consciously learn what others may "pick up" on their own and if we do not make the efforts to teach students strategies for processing extended discourse, they may be left behind. We may lose those who are not naturally talented but capable of learning this level of language.

A top–down progression of skills has been discussed: learning a way to approach the reading of expository chapters, of short stories and novels; learning how to comprehend and produce paragraphs with a clear understanding of the topic versus the "point," and appreciation of various types of paragraphs matched to the writer's purpose; learning to identify signals for cohesion in order to attend to and understand meaning connections; learning to decombine statements into single, more processable one-thought sentences and then to notice the relationships among those thoughts, that is, why they are in the same statement and what words connect them; learning to identify the three parts of questions (topic, facts, directions) and to formulate answers responsive to the direction words. Finally we discussed the needs of students who have difficulty at the word level of language. Some may be able to read words aloud but not realize that they do not know the meaning of those words. Some may naturally identify many unknown words because of their insufficient vocabulary knowledge. Both groups need to learn how to learn new words and need more than the typical assignment to find definitions and match to words. In addition to those who do not notice unfamiliar words and those who notice but do not know enough words, there are students who notice words but are less aware of or competent with syllables and sounds. They are "whole worders" who do not, naturally, notice the patterns within words. They need to be directed to the fine differences at the syllable level; to be engaged in discovery of shared patterns within words, in collecting example words with those patterns, in sorting words by patterns and in spelling words by shared patterns. Many adolescents and adults have persistent and serious spelling difficulty. Discussion focused on strategies for using spell checkers effectively and for improving spelling.

As in most teaching/learning experiences, it is critical that students be asked to explain and demonstrate knowledge of new language processing strategies to verify they understand and to cause active memory storage in their own words. When possible, the strategies need to be provided for and encouraged within the context of classrooms to establish habits for skills which are not natural and must be consciously learned. The goal of this effort is to ensure that students with insufficient language ability for extended discourse are not simply left to languish; that they are kept in the "language club" (Smith, 1988) and are taken beyond the conversational level of language with direct instruction and guided practice of needed skills.

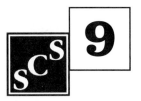

Using the Approach with Different Populations and in Different Settings

The shoulder-to-shoulder collaborative approach focused on problem solving is applicable within a variety of populations in a variety of settings. Our discussion thus far has featured language processing challenges and how to deal with them which can be an issue for many adolescents. This chapter discusses implications for adolescents within different diagnostic categories affecting language processing and within a variety of service delivery settings.

■□ ADOLESCENTS WITH TRAUMATIC BRAIN INJURY

Adolescents with a history of head trauma present differently according to the extent and character of their specific injuries, their pre-trauma histories, their personalities, family support and other issues. Adolescents with attention deficits also vary widely in the profiles they present, but there are similarities in these two groups of youngsters allowing us to consider them together. Impaired executive functions have been posed as a possible shared characteristic or "core of the disability" in both groups affecting self-awareness, ability to set goals, to make appropriate plans, to monitor the plans, and to strategically revise the plans (Ylvisaker & DeBonis, 2000). The shoulder-to-shoulder problem solving approach seems to address the areas of difficulty characteristic of executive function disability and to offer appropriate intervention strategies for these two groups of adolescents.

Establishing the Shoulder-to-Shoulder Approach

The shoulder-to-shoulder approach can be established using the tools discussed in Chapter 5. Adolescents should be given a chance at independently answering questions in the various interviews, of course, but it may be helpful or necessary for family members to fill out the same questionnaires to reflect their observations of the adolescent's language and learning so that contrasting perspectives can be considered and discussed. Adolescents whose views are widely disparate from those of their relatives may need help in clearly understanding themselves or in appreciating the difference in the way they present to others. Questions can be confusing or too abstract and may need to be restated in relation to a real life scenario to make them meaningful to many adolescents.

> *Think about sitting in a classroom when the teacher is teaching a new and difficult concept. Now think of your favorite teacher. What did he or she do to help you learn something new? What do you wish teachers would do to help you now?*

Clarifying Goals

The shoulder-to-shoulder problem solving collaboration can help youngsters with head trauma or attention problems discuss and clarify goals if their collaborators provide appropriate scaffolding to eliminate tangential thinking; to appreciate the abilities necessary to meet these goals when the proper questions are asked and information is found; and to compare these needed abilities to their own strengths and weaknesses revealed throughout the collaboration. If the adolescent has unrealistic expectations, this kind of discussion can be helpful for establishing realistic goals, identifying obstacles and planning interventions. In this kind of collaboration, of course, students may be unwilling to relinquish goals that seem too ambitious to their adult collaborator, but they may begin to understand how hard they will have to work and what they will need to do, specifically, to attain these goals. With supportive guidance and good information, the adolescent may surprise the adult by making up in tenacity what he or she lacks in actual abilities.

Checking Understanding and Feelings

The students, in this collaboration, need to restate in their own words, what has been discovered and discussed about their language and learning at all stages in the collaboration, including their understanding of results of formal and informal testing, of plans that have been made, and specific accommodations needed to implement the plan successfully. This comprehension or agreement check is important in all collaborations, but can be particularly critical when adolescents have had head trauma or attention problems interfering with taking in information. They may not have actively processed all that occurred within discussions or could have misconstrued what had been said. It is important for the student to explain the specific plans developed, of course, but it is equally important for them to explain the reasons for each part of the plan and to express their feelings about the plan. In order to make the necessary commitment to implementing plans that have been made it is critical that adolescents' feelings be thoroughly explored. One cannot assume, without their restating in their own words, that adolescent partners have heard what was said, understood what was said and have consciously chosen to participate in the plans. If the student cannot clearly explain the ideas discussed in the collaboration, he or she may not have understood what transpired in problem solving discussions. It is also possible that they have understood but do not have adequate expressive language skills for explaining. Comprehension checks with a collaborative partner clarifying and restating information as a model throughout the process followed by the student's restatement can provide productive practice to enable students to explain what they know about themselves and their needs. This step in the process cannot be overlooked.

■□ ADOLESCENTS WITH ATTENTION PROBLEMS

Students with attention problems clearly need to understand how they process and participate within communication and learning situations. Those with hyperactivity need to discover through collaboration with an adult, the impulsivity underlying their way of proceeding, (Barkley, ASHA 1998) where, when and how their impulsive style interferes in their learning or relationships and what might be done. Whether they take medicine to aid their attention or not, students with hyperactivity need to understand themselves as learners, to be engaged in active, guided reflection within problem solving, and to learn to work with others on their own behalf.

Collaborating with Students without Hyperactivity

Those without hyperactivity need the same opportunities to collaborate for better self-knowledge and problem solving. Without this kind of guided self-study, they may know as little about themselves as they do about what has transpired in class when their attention interferes. These adolescents need to work with an adult within a respectful shoulder-to-shoulder arrangement to develop a list of strengths and weaknesses, to make plans for self-monitoring of attention, and for revising plans to make them work. They need to learn what they can do on their own and to recognize when they need help to maintain adequate attention. Without this kind of joint exploration and planning, students with attention problems may not clearly understand what ADD or ADHD means in their life and learning. Without this awareness, they may not be able to do anything about it. The shoulder-to-shoulder, problem solving process should enable students to understand this diagnostic label of attention deficit in a general sense and to appreciate what they might share with others under that same category. They must also know about and be able to explain their own unique version of attention deficit. They should become experts, in the shoulder-to-shoulder collaboration, in the way they process information in conversations and for learning—what they might miss and under what conditions. Discussions provoked in the learning interview, mini-class interviews, and/or about daily school assignments may provide ongoing opportunities for this kind of self-discovery, particularly when time is provided for reflecting and self-reporting to show developing awareness of their language and learning (see Box 9–1).

BOX 9–1: *Questions for Discussion Regarding Attention*

1. When do I have the most trouble paying attention in class?
   (a) After the first 15 minutes, the last part of class?
   (b) When the teacher is talking for a long time?
   (c) When I do not understand and then "drift"?
2. What have I tried for better attention at these times?
3. What could I try?

■ ADOLESCENTS WITH BEHAVIOR PROBLEMS

Adolescents with behavior problems certainly need to collaborate with others to better understand themselves and their experiences, to appreciate good decisions in planning, and to anticipate the consequences of the plans they or others make. Informal interviews described in Chapter 5 may be less threatening or confrontational for this group of youngsters if conducted within a trust relationship than academic test questions, and may be more helpful than standardized scores. The adult, in these informal interviews, asks questions designed to elicit the adolescent's observations and opinions rather than asking questions that set up uncomfortable comparisons to more successful students with a greater store of accumulated formal knowledge. Problems identified in a shoulder-to-shoulder exploration are, presumably, personally relevant to the adolescent and may offer a successful way to invite the troubled youngster into productive collaboration. The adolescent with behavior problems may be amenable to investing in plans that they have helped devise for solving problems, that they have identified within the collaborative process with a supportive adult.

Communicating about Conflicts

Charlann Simon (personal communication, 1991) reported that seven of the eight middle school students being disciplined on a particular day at the school where she taught were her students with known language and learning problems. In her effort to understand why her students were the predominant group in this predicament, Simon concluded that they could not adequately explain what had occurred in an altercation. They could not tell "their side of it" and, as a result, were more likely to be punished than were their more articulate counterparts. Simon devised a way of collaborating with the students to help them better understand, explain and problem solve for conflict situations. She convinced the school to adopt her form (see Box 9–2) for use in the discipline process and she taught her students how to communicate the ideas needed for using this form. With this creative language intervention, these students were less often found in the discipline room.

Using this system for helping students explain their part in a dispute provides a good example for working with students to identify a specific problem (their inability to explain what had happened in an altercation), to devise a plan directed at that problem (learning and practicing appropriate responses for the discipline question form) and then to implement the plan within the needed situation (generalizing practiced responses to real discipline situations in which this form was used).

Asking Questions in Class

It seems likely that these same students may also have had difficulty asking questions or in formulating answers in academic classes, problems that could be revealed in the learning interview. If this were the case, one could teach them to respond appropriately within a particular situation (gaining clarification of new concepts presented in class)

BOX 9–2: *Communication Questionnaire (Simon, 1991)*

Name_____Date_____Grade_____
Age____

  I. Statement of reason for punishment.
 II. Opinion about the fairness of being punished.
III. Sequence of events that led to punishment.

             My version   The "other" version

1._____ 1._____
2._____ 2._____
3._____ 3._____
4._____ 4._____
5._____ 5._____

 IV. Problem-solving considerations.
     A. Event
     B. Communication
  V. Improvements based upon this experience—suggestions.

              My own   "The system"

1._____ 1._____
2._____ 2._____

---

with an appropriate, conscious strategy ("Tell what you know first and then ask about the specific idea about which you are unsure. Let's practice."). Matching interventions to the specific scenarios in which the problems occur seems a very practical way to establish problem solving approaches with adolescents. When the adult partner can elicit through discussion or observe directly real life situations in which the student spontaneously demonstrated telling what they knew first and then asked for specific information, the transfer to academic situations can be practiced but with the students' appreciation of the validity of this approach. It is always helpful to "catch" the student doing the right thing, label it and then practice it consciously.

Using Graphic Organizers for a Variety of Problems

Whitmire (2000) cited a case study in which the SLP used graphic organizers successfully with a student for improved reading and writing. This idea was then extended to problem solving involving the student's interpersonal conflicts, to a variety of other classroom learning tasks and used within personal counseling. The visual representation probably helped the student more clearly understand the plan and to think it through (warm up) before the stressful or new situations presented themselves. The SLP and her adolescent collaborator had found a good plan that fit this young woman's learning style and worked within a variety of problem areas.

Judging and Planning for Level of Difficulty

Adolescents with behavior problems pose special challenges within a problem solving approach. They may have a "short fuse" for struggle and give up or become angry when they cannot immediately make themselves clear in explaining a problem, for instance, or they may become discouraged just as quickly when solutions are not successful on the first trial. Many students with attention deficit also have these same problems with patience, although they might not distinguish themselves by acting out. In any case, students with this profile need extensive guided practice in using the traffic light analogy to judge their "level of knowing" and/or the difficulty of tasks to help them avoid viewing every problem or solution equally. They need help in learning to react differently to "red" issues (Concepts or plans that are difficult and require help from another person to even understand them), "yellow" issues, (Tasks that they can complete on their own, but require extended time and effort), as contrasted with "green" tasks or information that can be completed or understood independently and quickly. Promoting and guiding this classifying of problems and plans using traffic signal colors to acknowledge various levels of difficulty can be the main focus in a collaboration with an adolescent with behavior problems. Youngsters may learn, through this process, to select problems or goals that are "do-able" and allow them to achieve success. It is important that we intervene in this way to undo negative early learning experiences. Paul's (1991) finding that early learning problems were typical for many in the prison populations makes it imperative to reverse these failures in adolescents at risk by teaching and monitoring the use of effective strategies.

Creating a Successful Classroom

Bauer, Lynch and Murphy (1993) identified a teacher of those with "intensive severe behavior" problems (p. 15) that precluded their being placed in regular education classes. This teacher was known for her success with difficult classes so an ethnographic study was conducted to find out why she seemed to do well when others struggled with these youngsters. This teacher, the study found, adopted a "guidance approach" that stressed the facilitation of more effective communication and conventional behaviors rather than emulating the more controlling "authoritative-based classrooms" these students had previously experienced (p. 14). The teacher seemed to have strong feelings to guide her interactions with students: "each individual is responsible for his or her actions, each student is special and has strengths, and each student should be dealt with at his or her level." (p. 17) These views seem consistent with a shoulder-to-shoulder stance. This teacher established quickly, through her comments to students early in the school year, the belief that no one could make them follow rules and that they would have to decide on their own behavior. She clearly established and stated the rules ("the box"), but the students had to decide on their own to follow the rules. Students were responsible, for instance, for selecting appropriate partners and places for play, those that would not result in problems. The teacher required that students explain altercations beginning with the word "I" to focus on their own role in problems rather than to spend most of their time blaming others. She stressed her role as a co-participant by sharing her own experiences (using the "I" rule established to focus on one's own problems). She seemed to establish a shoulder-to-shoulder feeling through mutual respect and stress on self-management. The descriptions of this class suggested that the teacher and students were "in it together"; that she had a definite role in establishing an appropriate environment through clear rules, but that students had choices to make. She made the rules and routines very explicit, even physically acting them out at times and reviewed the pertinent rules before an activity to ensure understanding and memory during the first part of the year. She also taught new strategies in response to students' reporting of specific problems. This was referred to by the authors of this study as "new tool salesmanship." This seemed a good example of the student partner presenting the problem and the teacher then teaching them new strategies. One has to assume that at the beginning of a problem solving collaboration many adolescents do not have an adequate repertoire of appropriate and effective strategies to draw upon. This teacher regularly helped them add to their "bag of tricks" for problem solving.

Establishing Effective Classroom Communications

Bauer and colleagues (1993) concluded that this teacher established effective classroom communications primarily through honesty and clarity based on her strong understanding of her own personal goals. She was clear about what she expected and about her own role in the relationship with the students. Her actions were always consistent with her stated goals and she always reinforced self-direction, personal responsibility, the value of individuals and the importance of support. She made the rules and routines explicit and, presumably, the students knew how to proceed in this classroom. Finally, she helped the students learn new "tools." When they made the personal decisions to follow the routines and rules, then this teacher played her part appropriately and helped them learn new productive behaviors. She demonstrated, for example, fifteen instances of "new tool salesmanship" within the first three days of school, this teacher showing early on that she could help them with their difficulties in specific, responsive ways.

Sharing Responsibility with Youngsters

A shoulder-to-shoulder, problem solving approach may be achieved best with youngsters with behavior disorders when the adult takes major responsibility for establishing a workable and fair "box" as the teacher above did; establishes the "I" rule that requires participants to focus on their own problems and plans, when rules and routines are made very clear with reminders as needed and students' roles in decision making very gradually increased toward a more equal collaboration. Students with a long history of being the "bad guys" may need to experience the positive effects of another's structure before they can contribute significantly to designing their own structure, but they should have some role from the beginning, even it if is simply choosing from alternative aspects of a structure. Perhaps the teacher's providing tools for dealing with students' reported problems helped establish personal motivation to engage in this joint problem solving process from the beginning because they learned something helpful early in the process.

Facilitating the Shoulder-to-Shoulder Approach

A shoulder-to-shoulder problem solving approach can work best for behavior problems when everyone understands their roles in the process and understands the usual routine for joint problem solving sessions; when there is agreement about how plans will be implemented and about how success will be judged (see Box 9–3). Finally, success depends on students' being able to explain the structure for the collaboration in their own words and on the structure being reinforced appropriately to establish an effective routine. A written contract may be an effective way of summing up for making the structure clear especially for students who may not understand or trust a new relationship with an adult.

They may need to see what they will be asked to do.

BOX 9–3: *Factors in Facilitating Shoulder-To-Shoulder*

1. Roles are clear and understood.
2. Routine for joint problem solving is clear.
3. There is agreement about how plans will be implemented and judged.
4. Adolescent can explain the structure for the collaboration.
5. A written contract may be necessary for clarity and trust.

■☐ ADOLESCENTS WITH SPEECH FLUENCY PROBLEMS

The shoulder-to-shoulder problem solving approach seems consistent with the typical work of SLPs and adolescents who stutter. SLPs have collaborated with young clients to help them discover exactly what they do when they are speaking fluently and when they are dysfluent. Shames and Florance (1980), for instance, describe an interviewing process important to their collaboration with clients having fluency problems. Johnson and Heinze (1994) provide a fluency questionnaire that elicits information about adolescents' interests, attitudes about school and specific information about speech. Such interviews allow adolescents to think about and present what they know about their speech and, coupled with story swapping, can encourage reporting of pertinent experiences, reveal the adolescent's point of view, and provide a language sample.

Involving the Adolescent in their Intervention

Adolescents with fluency difficulty are not always but can be included in the development of therapy plans. SLPs typically check the client's understanding of recommended strategies for increasing fluency. We involve them in monitoring their experiences and evaluating their success in implementing therapy plans. The problem solving approach— define and narrow the problem, make a plan and implement it, then evaluate and revise the plan—seems to apply well to this population. The shoulder-to-shoulder quality which stresses the responsibility and value of each partners' contribution also seems helpful in avoiding the "laying on of the hands" expectations of adolescents who may put all their hopes in adults' making and effecting plans to "fix" their speech problems. In order to ensure the active engagement of the adolescent client, the SLP may need to present a variety of ways to achieve fluency, to allow the adolescent to select a technique and to explain their choice of "plans." Daly (1988) stresses the adolescent client's need to know that the clinician has a good plan that they believe in and that this plan has been successful in helping others. In some cases, then, the adolescent's role within the problem solving may be focused more appropriately on understanding and being able to explain a plan chosen by the adult along with an active part in evaluating his or her success with and helping to revise the plan as needed. Daly (1988) reminds us of an old adage that we "speak not only to tell others what we think but to tell ourselves what we think too" (p. 13), which makes the collaborative, problem solving productive for adolescents to explain and inform the process and to understand themselves.

■□ HELPING ADOLESCENTS WITH PRAGMATIC LANGUAGE PROBLEMS

The reference to acceptable sentence making in Hymes (1971) provides a good description of pragmatic language "rules" understood by many and the need for appropriate interaction of adolescents both in and out of school. Knowing "who can say what, in what way, where, and when, by what means and to whom" (p.15) can provide a guideline for exploring and understanding social language strengths and weaknesses. Adolescents can collect and report anecdotes showing situations in which they felt successful or unsuccessful in their communication attempts. When there are problems they can decide with the help of their collaborator if the problem focused on their talking at the wrong time or place, about the wrong topic, using the wrong style, being wrong to say what they did, or saying it to the wrong person. In the effort to understand how to make a good plan to right their wrong communication, the adolescent can be asked to observe their peers for just the aspect of conversation they need to learn. Reporting their observations, further discussing the situation with an adult or within a small group and then practicing skills within a role play fits into the shoulder-to-shoulder, problem solving approach.

Using Grice's Postulates to Guide Problem Solving

Adolescents can also learn about the guiding rules that Grice (1975) postulated to help them identify problems and make appropriate plans. 1) Making your comment just informative enough can be taught and practiced using the old–new balance principle and observation of the adult collaborator as listener followed by observation within peer interactions, of teachers and students in class. Students need practice in watching to determine when their listener is confused or understands and wants to move on to new information. The adolescent who regularly shows off by telling more than is required causing a groan from his or her peers comes to mind along with the overly succinct, "bottom-line" style of many students who say the bare minimum and need to learn to elaborate in some situations. 2) Grice's second principle to be sincere or truthful can be addressed within a collaboration with students who exaggerate to seek approval or those who do not recognize when someone is violating this principle to tease or make a joke. Adolescents who understand that sincerity is the "default feature" of normal conversation can then be directed to try to figure out what people do to indicate that they are violating the principle. Adolescents who don't "get" jokes or don't realize that someone is teasing them often cause their family to stop joking or teasing, so they need direct help to develop awareness of this kind of language. Identifying this as a problem can allow adult collaborators to demonstrate teasing, dry humor, over exaggerating for effect, and so forth. 3) The third principle, relevance, is critical for helping students learn how to introduce and maintain topics. This can be identified, and strategies devised and practiced within the collaboration, through assigned field experiments for observing and practicing with peers. Conversations on paper can be an effective way to show concretely where and how topics were introduced, maintained and changed. 4) The final postulate, "be clear," is implemented throughout the shoulder-to-shoulder, problem solving effort. Adults model and guide adolescents in clarifying through well-ordered and appropriately concise statements. The restatement of problems and plans that is a regular requirement for good communication in this approach provides extensive practice for this principle.

Practicing Strategies for Needed Language

The need for adults to clearly understand as evident by follow-up questions in the various interviews and within problem defining and planning in the ongoing collaboration seems to encourage the explicitness that characterizes expository discourse (Wallach & Miller, 1988). The story swapping or reporting of observed situations included in this approach helps adolescents practice and develop their narrative language. Students engaged in problem solving, even within a one-on-one collaboration are practicing many of the specific language skills needed in classrooms including appropriate questioning, turntaking, and providing appropriate information (Ehren, 1994). Adolescents with pragmatic language problems seem particularly appropriate for the shoulder-to-shoulder approach because their lack of social skill often interferes and stops their communication development. They either assume the style of a newcomer and disappear in class and in social situations because of their lack of communication or they interact inappropriately and alienate others with inappropriate communication. Either way, someone needs to focus on pragmatics with these adolescents. Small group collaboration seems most appropriate to allow for a variety of observations replicating, to a certain extent, what might happen both in social and in classroom situations. Ehren (1994) stresses the need to focus on the "how-to's" or strategies for improved language which are critical with pragmatic language. The *Skillstreaming* books (Goldstein & McGinnis, 1997) provide for identifying problems, practicing strategies within role playing and then within classroom or small group activities and, presumably, discussing and practicing the "how to's" more thoroughly in role playing again, if necessary. Plans made in response to problem solving in the approach suggested in this book require that adults and adolescents discover, model and practice specific strategies for solving problems.

■□ PROBLEM SOLVING IN SMALL GROUP SETTINGS

There may be adolescents who need small group sessions to best iden-tify their problems, to understand the roles in collaboration ("You give me your best guess and then I'll help") to react freely to their collabo-rators' observations, and to contribute ideas for planning, evaluating and revising plans. They can learn strategies from others in the small group, and may need a slower pace or less competitive nature in this setting as compared with whole class participation. Other students' comments in the small group can facilitate thinking and commenting, sometimes in ways that adults cannot in individual intervention.

■□ PROVIDING NEEDED INDIVIDUAL INTERVEN-TION

There are always students who need individual sessions for self-discovery, modeling and practicing of strategies. Those who are learn-ing how to manage academic language while also trying to acquire new content can require extensive, individually guided practice for understanding paragraphs, complex statements and questions, for dealing with unknown and specialized vocabulary, for planning and implementing writing strategies, and for dealing with spelling issues interfering with writing and self-esteem. The extra examples and prac-tice required for language learning can be difficult within a classroom where many others are ready to move at a faster pace. Individual help along with classroom reinforcement and accommodations can enable the adolescent to participate optimally within the whole group.

■□ WORKING WITH AT RISK STUDENTS IN THE CLASSROOM SETTING

In addition to the individual preparation, at risk students can and should work within classrooms. Teachers can provide for practice in specific language processing strategies within classroom routines in ways that are essential for those with special needs and helpful to many other students. Regularly introducing or reviewing important concepts by engaging the class in sentence decombining to focus on each important thought to be learned can emphasize the content for everyone while also providing language processing practice. Asking students to gain extra credit for successfully estimating test grades and/or to predict which test questions they might miss by "dotting" them may be important for adolescents with attention problems and for all who need help in "owning" their own learning. The same is true if teachers require students to decombine test questions and/or to "cor-rect" wrong answers by supplying appropriate questions to match those answers. These strategies must be taught and practiced individually for some students but can be helpful to many if implemented in the classroom. Teachers who are willing to integrate them into their regular lessons for at risk students may discover their benefit to all students and become enthusiastic collaborators. .

■ SUMMARY

The intent, "flavor" and implementation of the shoulder-to-shoulder, problem solving collaborative approach seems clearly applicable to a variety of different populations of adolescents within a variety of service delivery models. The fostering of problem identifying and solving, of self-monitoring and appreciating one's role and responsibility within joint collaboration seems possible and desirable in many situations designed for adolescents with special needs in language and learning. There may be times when a one-on-one collaboration is necessary along with reinforcement of strategies within classroom situations. There may be times, for example, to identify problems and practice pragmatic language strategies, when small group work is best. There may be other times when this approach works within large groups with the support of the collaborators in planning. In any of these settings, with adolescents in different diagnostic categories, problem solving is necessary and well-served within a shoulder-to-shoulder approach.

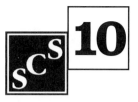

Transitions— Understanding Needs and Advocating for Accommodations for Post-secondary Schooling and Employment

Actively engaging adolescents throughout high school in the planning of and periodic review of their Individual Educational Plans (IEPs) is important. Ensuring that they can explain their goals and educational accommodations is even more important. Adolescents may not always want to be included in group planning meetings with many adults talking about them, but someone needs to ensure that they are informed, that they contribute to, understand and agree with their educational plans, and that they have a role in assessing progress whenever possible. It seems clear that adolescents' understanding of and support for their learning plans in high school will help prepare them for transitioning to higher learning or to the world of work. Gee (1996) asks educators to consider to "what sort of social group do I intend to apprentice the learner?" (p. 44) as guiding adolescents to be more informed about themselves as learners can enable them to eventually join a broader range of groups.

■□ WORKING WITH ADOLESCENTS FOR TRANSITIONS

Those working with adolescents at transition periods, going into post-secondary education or into the work force can certainly engage students using the shoulder-to-shoulder approach, and this seems to describe what vocational counselors typically do. They inform at risk students of vocational options and guide their planning beginning in eighth grade. If students are then regularly asked to explain these options, the pros and cons of various plans, their preferences for possible plans and their reasons for their own preferences, their understanding and participation can be better assessed (see Box 10–1). Eighth graders guided to know themselves and to problem solve through the shoulder-to-shoulder approach have a good start in confronting the challenges of higher-level classes and employment. Those anticipating college or technical schools certainly need to understand the requirements of these programs considered in light of their abilities. Intellectual, academic and vocational aptitude testing provides material for discussion and planning. Speakers, mentoring programs, and brochures can be helpful if adolescents are guided in explaining what they understand and how it fits into their plans. Adolescents can be guided in explaining aloud or in writing their understanding of their strengths and weaknesses for school and employment, their goals and their plans. The individual educational plans that follow a student with special needs should be accompanied by an audiotape or written account by the student showing their participation and understanding of themselves as learners and potential employees at transitions from middle school to high school and at the end of high school.

Checking Comprehension of Language Learning Needs and Plans

Jan, the young girl (See Chapter 4) who seemed to be listening but then could not report what had been said, offered an important lesson to those collaborating with adolescents. Neither she nor I realized that she was not really processing and comprehending what was being discussed. Jan and many adolescents who share her listening style, need others to check their understanding and to help them appreciate the need for this checking.

Comprehension checks can be a critical element in an educational or vocational plan particularly when adolescents have language limitations. At these comprehension checks, It is imperative that students

---

BOX 10–1: *My Transition Plan*

At this transition time my strengths based on schoolwork, testing, discussions with others and my own observations are as follows:

_____

_____

_____

_____

I understand that my weaker areas are as follows:

_____

_____

_____

_____

To do my best work I need the following kind of help from others: _____

_____

To do my best work I need to do the following things for myself:

_____

_____

The professions that interest me now are _____

_____

_____

To be a good candidate for these kinds of work I will need to do the following this next year:

_____

_____

---

restate *in their own words* their understanding of the problems, goals and plans. This restating can provide a way for youngsters to feel ownership in personalized problem solving, can reveal mismatches between their understandings and others' and can provide practice in accurately explaining and advocating for themselves. Because their being able to effectively advocate for themselves is important for success in post-secondary education and within their careers, adolescents need many opportunities to practice the oral presentation of their own educational needs and plans.

Checking Comprehension Requires an Aggressive Approach

Adults and the adolescents themselves may assume that they have processed what has been seen and heard in a class, in an educational planning session or within an ongoing collaboration simply because they were present, but there is a need for aggressive checking of understanding when there are language problems. The typical, "Is everyone with me?" or "Does anyone have a question?" will not reveal what has actually been heard, understood and stored by adolescents. One cannot assume that a youngster has actively processed and internalized information unless there is 1) a regular time for checking understandings and agreements; 2) a required restating or writing of the understandings; and 3) the student's feelings about the plans have also been explored.

Checking Comprehension Includes Noting Verbal and Nonverbal Messages

The restating of what has been said, an active listening style, has long been promoted for counselors, teachers and parents as a good way to communicate (Rogers, 1942; Ginott, 1971; Gordon, 1976, Andrews & Summers, 1988) and adults should also periodically check their own understanding of the younger collaborators' comments with restatements in their own words. Andrews and Summers (1988) remind us to reflect in our restatements not just the verbal but also nonverbal communications to allow for exploration of underlying feelings. If, for instance, a youngster can explain his or her educational plan adequately but body language indicates a lack of interest in or agreement with the plan, this issue needs to be discussed.

In a case study reported by Feeney and Ylvisaker (1995), a high school student with traumatic brain injury had collaborated with an SLP, a psychologist and teachers to identify goals and to decide on the support that would be needed to improve behavior and academic success. The student learned to create graphic organizers for complex academic tasks and helped monitor the effects of this and other accommodations on his school performance. This student apparently understood and appreciated his plan and also learned something about advocating because he, later, successfully negotiated with his supervisor the use of this same accommodation on a new job.

Understanding Why Adolescents Require Comprehension Checks

Some adolescents with a history of language or learning problems have never requested information about their periodic testing or about the accommodations that have been made for them. They may have left everything to their teachers and parents up to this time because of a lack of interest. Others have not been invited into the process and have little of the information others know about them as learners. In the effort to establish their needs and to obtain appropriate help in classrooms, the adults may have forgotten to assess the students' understanding or personal investment in the process. Still other students may have been curious but found it embarrassing to discuss their language or learning problems. A fourth group of adolescents may have lacked the communication skill for participating fully in discussions of their testing, observations of classroom learning and/or their IEPs. A final group of adolescents may be focused on just getting out of school, without appreciating the realities of life beyond school and the benefits of self-knowledge. Regardless of the reasons, adolescents who do not know their own needs may have difficulty advocating for themselves on the job or in post-secondary classes.

SLPs Helping Adolescents at Transitions to Post-secondary Schooling

Speech-language pathologists can be instrumental in preparing students for transitions by assessing and documenting persistent language problems with both standardized testing and clinical observations, by helping students appreciate their strengths and limitations in language and the implications for school learning, by guiding practice in explaining language and learning needs, in asking for assistance with knowledge of the specific kind of help needed, and in helping students decide upon realistic educational and career goals. In this effort, the SLP and the student can focus on the IEP with many restatings on the student's part, both in oral and in written form to show understanding and for practice in expression. This activity also provides opportunities to explore varied ways to explain for different listeners (professors, roommates, friends, employers), provides practical reasons to expand vocabulary with the student's first writing or telling in a conversational style and then, with help, considering specific vocabulary that may be more clear or appropriate. The SLP's role seems critical also for explaining the impact of language problems to others on a transition team, particularly when the student's speech is clear and skills are adequate for short interchanges but not for processing academic language. Everyone, including the student, needs to appreciate that college and career success require extended discourse beyond the short interchanges of conversation, and appropriate planning depends on this understanding. The SLP can be a consultant within a college support program engaging in interdisciplinary collaboration, can continue to provide language remediation focused on notetaking, strategies for completing written assignments in class and for interpreting and presenting ideas in class discussion, three skills college faculty noted as difficult for the language learning disordered (LLD) students (Schneider, Philips, & Ganschow, 2000) and can serve on committees petitioning for special accommodations. (Ganschow, Philips & Schneider, 2001).

Using Accommodations in Post-Secondary Schooling

Adolescents and their collaborators need to know what accommodations are appropriate and available. Aune and Friehe (1996) have discussed accommodations in three categories: those to be implemented in class by the student with instructor agreement; those to be provided primarily by the instructor; and those that can be arranged by support services. Simon (2001) speaks of auxiliary aids and services as con-

trasted with academic adjustments as two categories of accommodations. Aaron and Baker (1991) delineate self-help strategies to be
employed by the students themselves as compared with help from
"external sources" including a "mentor tutor" and academic tutors. The
mentor tutor's role seems similar to that of the LD coordinator
mentioned by Ganschow, Phillips and Schneider (2001). It can be helpful to think of who, where, when, and how needed services can be deliv-
ered and these various models can guide that planning (see Box 10–2).

Working with Professors

Some college support programs have worked with professors in developing classroom communication strategies effective for those with language learning problems. The content enhancement model (Lenz,
Bulgren & Hudson, 1990) can be helpful in working with these professors. It includes routines to orient students to the topic (warming up)
and devices to facilitate understanding including extra examples, clear
comparisons, highlighting cause–effect relationships; devices for storing and remembering information (associations, rhyming, loci, key
words, etc.), and devices for organizing information (Ehren, 1994).
Landmark College, a post-secondary setting for those with learning
difficulties, provides teaching principles. These principles ask instructors in their study skills program: 1) to begin at point zero, that is, the
appropriate starting point for students; 2) to break complex tasks into
micro-units to allow for better processing; 3) to use a multi-sensory
approach; 4) to model for students; and 5) to teach to automatization.
(Baucom, Cole, Denny, Hinckley, & Villemaire, 1993).

Making Clear the Responsibilities of Students

It is important to clarify the role of the students at transitions. Nelson
(1994) reminded us that the success of students with language learning
disabilities in post-secondary education or in a job depends on the "independent skills, coping mechanisms, and strategies that the individual
acquires" during prior schooling. Students must understand their needs
and the accommodations required. Bashir, Goldhammer and Bigaj (2000)
describe a six step program for helping a graduate student with LLD
toward self-determination through self-knowledge and better communication: 1) reviewing assessments and determining a profile of needs and
strengths; 2) making a commitment to the process; 3) developing better
communication; 4) enhancing self-knowing regarding the impact of
communication problems; 5) using strategies to work with self-beliefs;
and 6) integrating risk taking with independence (p. 56).

Students must be able to explain their needs and strategies that
have previously worked for them—to their friends, roommates, tutors,
advisors and to their instructors. They may be required to deliver

BOX 10–2: *Accommodation Options*

(Aaron & Baker, 1991, Aune & Friehe, 1996; Ganschow, Philips, &
Schneider, 2001; Bauer & Tutonis, 1996; Simon, J.A. 2001)

- Extended time (quizzes, test, lab work, in-class writing)
- Test questions read aloud or read and restated
- Student paraphrases test questions before answering
- Tests taken in a quiet area
- Reformatted exams
- Oral tests—questions and answers
- Scribes for writing answers on tests or for in-class writing
- Test error analysis to determine problems
- Advanced notice of oral reading or oral presentation in class
- Advanced copies of overheads, lecture outlines
- Study guides (in person or through internet)
- Notetakers in class or copies of class and text notes
- Tape-recorded lectures
- Tape-recorded texts
- Using calculators and spell checkers in class.
- Preferential seating and placement within small group work
- Use of a personal amplification system
- Option for voluntary oral response in class
- Opportunity for questions at set times in class
- Experience/demonstration/visuals to augment lectures
- Explanations in known vocabulary and less complex sentences
- Slower rate of speech and/or pause at the end of a thought to allow processing. Asking for paraphrasing from students of major points to allow at risk students to reprocess and understand.
- Allowances for spelling and mechanics for in-class writing
- Permission to rewrite assignments
- Access to supplementary textbooks to allow reviewing topics in a different form or writing style
- Assistance in organizing information for writing or for study
- One-on-one meetings with professor at office hours
- E-mail communication with professor
- Visual cues to aid listening
- Taking a reduced class load (12 hours).
- Substituting less demanding courses without jeopardizing required knowledge

letters explaining their needs to professors. and to ask for specific accommodations such as help in identifying a fellow student to provide copies of their notes, to ask for permission to tape record lectures, and to request extended time for test taking, for written assignments in class and for completing lab work.

College students with language learning disorders listed accommodations they found most helpful and included the following: allowances for poor spelling on in-class writing, advance notice for lengthy reading assignments, extended time for multiple choice tests and for essay answers, having a copy of another student's notes, and testing in an undistracting place (Schneider, Philips, & Ganschow, 2000); students at transitions might find this information helpful.

Students must identify and explain their specific concerns about college classes and report problems in a timely manner to professors and support personnel. This is important for all college freshman but at risk students must be even more vigilant in obtaining appropriate help before they are too far behind in their work. Those working with students can facilitate this by scheduling meeting times with the understanding that the student's identifying of problems will be first on the agenda.

Students are responsible for using the services available and listed on their plan including meeting regularly and consistently with tutors, consulting professors during office hours and showing exemplary class attendance (Downey & Snyder, 2001). They may need to work on needed skills such as keyboarding to facilitate use of computers; on enhancing their awareness of their typical spelling errors to allow for independent proofreading; and use of a hand held spell checker for in-class writing. Students with language limitations may have to spend extra time previewing the next day's topic as a regular preparation for listening. Students also need to know that they are expected to operate within the social and behavioral rules for all students and a review of campus rules seems in order. Adolescents need to appreciate that they are entitled to accommodations and help but that others will naturally be more willing to help when they see that students are working to help themselves.

Students need to be clear on what services they are entitled to under the law and what the college is not required to do for them. For instance, colleges apparently do not have to provide specially trained tutors and may provide only what is available to all students, which could mean peer tutors, if that is what is available to other students (Simon, 2001). Students need to discuss these issues with their mentor tutor or LD coordinator in order to advocate appropriately for themselves. Asking students what they think the school is obligated to provide may reveal misunderstandings and allow for learning about the requirements.

Collaborating regarding Various Accommodations

Mentor tutors, advisors or LD coordinators need to help students with special needs select appropriate courses. Initially, they may want to

avoid the more abstract courses and/or professors who maintain a fast
pace and require extensive reading. Advisors may suggest that students register for 15 hours a semester with the assumption that 12
hours may be more appropriate. This advanced planning, however,
will allow a student to drop a course and make the schedule manageable. The student and the collaborator need to compose a letter to professors in which special needs and requests for accommodations are
made explicit. The adult partner in this collaboration may order
recorded textbooks, arrange for sign language interpreters, for braille
or large print materials, tape recorders or lap top computers, arrange
for academic tutors, arrange for the student to enroll in a study strategies course; guide the student in deciding on a weekly study schedule,
work goals and specific ways the student is to monitor the plan in
order to identify problems to be solved with the partner.

Working with Mentors or Tutors: One Approach

Those adolescents going beyond high school to higher education need
plans in place in order to do well. Some of the suggestions in this chapter may be helpful for all students transitioning from high school, but
are critical for those with special needs. After they have been accepted
into a program with an appropriate support system and have completed one week of class, students should schedule a study conference
with their adult collaborator: LD coordinator, mentor tutor, speech language pathologist, or academic tutor. The student should come to the
meeting with new textbooks, a syllabus or outline from every class and
a schedule of professors' office hours. The student and advisor plan a
study schedule on which they show all classes, tutoring sessions,
extracurricular activities, meal times and professor's office hours. They
review the syllabus for each class and transfer due dates for assignments and tests onto a calendar for review within weekly tutoring sessions. The tutor and student then plan scheduled times for reviewing
notes after each class, completing the reading and previewing for the
next class. They discuss what to do in those study periods—make a
"study script" (Review notes by reading aloud, filling in missing information while you remember it and then restating each note in your
words, skip over those you can't explain and ask someone else to
explain them. Preview reading and make a web showing the title and
subtitles, read the chapter summary then read each section or paragraph, if needed, and write a note showing the topic and the point
being made about the topic. Review previous class notes and your
reading notes before class).

The student meets again with the collaborator after one week of
trying out the study plan and study scripts to discuss what is working
and what has to be modified in the plan. The student needs to explain
and show what he/she is actually doing within each study period for
each subject to see what adjustments are needed. It is important for students to demonstrate reviewing class notes to check the accuracy of

their paraphrasing for comprehending, to show how they read or listen to a portion of text and make some notes to check their ability to identify "wheat from chaff." With these checks and appropriate modifications, the student can then try out the revised plan and meet with his or her major collaborator periodically or the academic tutor can take over the collaboration.

In regular academic tutoring sessions, a routine should be developed in which the student first explains any problems or potential problems identified in the past week. ("What's working, what isn't working, what is is bothering you?"). When the tutor explains a concept or possible modification to be made in studying, the student should, regularly, explain it back in his/her own words (tutor–tutee principle) to ensure understanding and facilitate storage of the information. At the end of a session, the student should summarize what has been done and what is important as a follow-up during study in the next week. With a good plan in place and collaborators to help, the students should be well informed and ready to problem solve his/her way through academic or technical college.

Tutoring as an Accommodation

Academic tutors are especially important for those with language difficulties to guide their study and ensure that the plan is effective. Deshler and Graham (1980) suggest that tutors knowledgeable in the course material are the appropriate ones to tape textbooks when word decoding problems or attention style prevent independent reading. The tutor can facilitate listening comprehension by providing an overview of a new chapter, by stressing or repeating important points, explaining concepts and terms, and finishing by including a summary of the chapter and review of the questions. There is often the suggestion that at risk students read along as they listen to taped texts, but students with severe decoding problems may find this difficult as may those who become overloaded by simultaneously reading and listening to academic language.

Tutors can guide students to proofread using the COPS acronym (capitals, organization, punctuation, spelling) (Wong & Wong, 1988). This approach assumes that students recognize the errors within the categories represented; however, those with significant problems may need to first work with tutors in collecting, grouping and naming their typical errors in writing (Neglecting the final 'S to show ownership, forgetting to indicate a proper name with a capital, not marking sentence "boundaries" with capital and ending punctuation, etc.) and to focus at first on only a few important errors in self-proofing with the tutor looking for the remaining mistakes. Many students may need to watch and listen as their tutor models the process many times and have extensive guided practice before they become good at identifying their own errors.

Helping Students Actively Process Text

Students with listening and reading comprehension problems may need extensive help in activating or building sufficient background information as a regular prereading step and in identifying main ideas. Tutors can regularly direct students to note the topic and to note the "point" being made about that topic in a paragraph. Tutors can also model, teach and implement with students the reciprocal teaching (Palinscar, 1986) approach that includes tutor and students taking turns clarifying the task, activating background information, determining main idea, evaluating content in light of prior information, checking comprehension and clarifying confusions, and making and testing conclusions.

Aaron and Baker discuss guidelines for tutors in working with at risk students, as shown in Box 10–3.

BOX 10–3: *Guidelines For Tutors (Adapted from Aaron & Baker, 1991)*

1. Assist students but do not do their work.
2. Appreciate the difference between language problems and intelligence.
3. Respect the students. Start with their understandings and build on them.
4. Focus on improving comprehension more than on word decoding.
5. Use positive but honest feedback as much as possible.
6. Practice active listening. Restating the student's comments is helpful for communication and provides models for translating intentions into language.
7. Understand and recognize different kinds of reading problems.
8. Remember that "tutoring is a cooperative venture." You create the environment that allows the students to do the work. However, they do the work and, when it works, it is because they are able to do it.

Using Technology to Aid in Writing

Technology to assist those with writing difficulty includes word processing with spell checkers and grammar checkers, special tools to support transcription, word prediction programs, speech synthesis and speech recognition, and hypermedia. Macarthur (2000) reviewed the limited research on these assistive devices and concluded that word processing can improve overall writing and help students learn to revise more effectively if there is instruction to support the technology.

Word prediction programs that anticipate words in writing have potential for those with severe spelling problems especially when the program provides synthesized speech for reading the predicted words. Macarthur (2000) noted that more research is needed to investigate ways to help students plan their writing and mentioned one effort in which a program included guiding questions before, during and after composing and helped high achieving sixth graders improve their writing (Salomon, 1992). For the disorganized and/or impulsive writer these questions can serve as reminders and increase reflection specifically directed to planning in writing.

Use of e-mail and the Internet has improved response to distant audiences in writing (Cohen & Riel, 1989), which might result in elaborated language to make the information clear to the reader. Hypermedia seems to motivate youngsters, but it is unclear what impact it has on the quality of writing. (Daiute & Morse, 1994; Bahr, Nelson & Van Meter (1996). In general the combination of instruction and technology seems to offer the most effective help to improve the writing of at risk students,

Helping Students Use Accommodations Effectively

Although he is discussing handwriting problems, Bain (1991) makes three important points about "compensatory devices" which seem applicable to many accommodations (Bain, Bailet & Moats, 1991). First, it should be clear to all involved that direct instruction and daily supervised practice are needed until there is student mastery of alternative strategies: word processing, use of a tape recorder, recorded texts, and so forth. There may be adolescents at transition times who have previously tried and rejected accommodations perhaps because there was no one to help them problem solve as they tried to become proficient in a new skill. The second point stresses that accommodations do not always completely substitute for a skill: handwriting, spelling, and so forth. Problem solving or direct teaching should not be abandoned too quickly for enhancing skills in this area in spite of learning accommodations. There may be situations in which the student has to be able to function passably without the accommodation and neither the students nor their instructors should assume that an accommodation will be completely successful. For instance, the poor speller may produce a correctly spelled homonym (there, for their) that will not be identified by many spell checkers so direct teaching of homonyms may be necessary. Misspellings can vary so much from the intended word that the spell check cannot select the intended word, so spelling may need to be remediated to the point where accommodations can work. Third, some accommodations may require the same skill that they are supposed to circumvent. For instance, some students with handwriting problems may be apraxic which can also adversely affect their keyboarding ability. Students with reading comprehension problems may also have difficulty understanding recorded textbooks presenting complex, expository language. Problems with accommodations can be identified with collaborative, ongoing problem solving and it is important not to assume accommodations will work automatically.

■□ ACCOMMODATING ADOLESCENTS WITHIN THE WORKPLACE

Adolescents entering the world of work have to know themselves, the requirements of the job they are seeking, what accommodations will be necessary, what the employer is required to do in accommodating special needs, and what seems appropriate in the current situation. If the requirements of IDEA have been met, the student has been guided in making a transition plan at the end of middle school, periodic comprehension checks have confirmed understanding and investment of the student, monitoring and problem solving have ensured compliance, then the transition from high school to work should be smooth. The transition team including the adolescent should have a good basis for selecting the level and kind of support needed to enter a workplace environment. Competitive employment requires training and supervision (apprenticeships, internships, on-the-job training or transitional employment) with ongoing problem solving and expectation that, with this kind of assistance, the adolescent or young adult should eventually be able to manage on his or her own . The term, supported employment, implies that continued help is needed including a student's being placed on the job in individual or small groups trained and supervised together, within a benchwork model in which people with disabilities complete contract work at a site away from the business, and/or the mobile crew model in which a team of workers moves from one job site to another with more support than in other models mentioned so far. Sheltered employment implies that the employee works best within a self-contained workplace where workers are trained and work on piecework jobs (Health Resource Center, 1992). One can see that the amount of accommodation varies according to the needs of the client, which determine the level of support required.

Analyzing Job Requirements

In addition to understanding their own needs, adolescents entering the job market need to understand what is required in various jobs. Job analysis involves collecting, organizing and evaluating information about a job. Physical factors such as lifting, standing or sitting for long periods, endurance for repetitive tasks, and so forth are worth investigating even when there are no overt physical limitations. The youngster who is easily bored, for instance, should know what he or she must do for extended periods. Environmental factors such as noise levels, hazards, ventilation, lighting, types of tools or equipment provide topics for discussion in collaborating with adolescents who are easily distracted, for instance, or those with allergies, those who are not well-coordinated or are impulsive and may need to reflect about using certain tools. Cognitive factors to be considered in a job can include the amount of and the rate at which information must be processed, attention requirements, new learning required, temporal and spatial orientation, sequential organization, flexibility, decision making, self-monitoring and initiative expected, judgment, academic levels for reading, writing, spelling, and so forth. Behavioral/interpersonal issues can include the ability to work independently, self-control, ability to cooperate and interact with others on a group goal, willingness to accept supervision, response to stress and frustration tolerance (Wachter, Fawber & Scott, 1987). Considering these issues can allow youngsters to better evaluate a job in spite of what seems like "good money," for instance, and can enable the collaborating partners to plan modifications as needed.

Understanding the Employers' Responsibilities

Lord-Larson and McKinley (1995) report that the Americans with Disabilities Act requires an employer to: 1) analyze the duties and purpose of a job; 2) discuss the potential employee's limitations or special need for accommodations; 3) identify the accommodations and determine how effective they will be for the potential employee; and 4) select appropriate accommodations available considering the preferences of the employee. Employers may have difficulty assessing job requirements in relation to every kind and level of need and may need extensive help from those who know the potential employee. If adolescents can clearly explain their needs this is an asset in working as it is in post-secondary education.

Helping Adolescents Communicate Their Needs for Accommodation on the Job

Assuming that adolescents have learned about themselves as learners and language users within a collaboration throughout their school years and also know what accommodations they need, there is a third, very important issue—being able to communicate this information effectively. It is helpful if the adolescent or young adult in question also knows general skills that are needed for good job performance such as being able to adapt to job demands, being motivated and self-directed, having effective interpersonal and communication abilities, being able to apply what he or she has learned in school, being able to manage personal and self-care needs, and being self-reliant about transportation (Gobble, Henry, Pfahl, & Smith, 1987). These same authors also give examples of specific work abilities and matching work situations that can guide discussions. They offer diagnostic questions that can help identify problems specific to the worker in question and the job to be done (see Box 10–4).

BOX 10–4: *Questions to Help Identify Problems On the Job*

(Gobble, Henry, Pfahl, & Smith, 1987)

1. How much time is required for the new worker to:
   (a) understand the task?
   (b) organize and plan the task?
   (c) to complete the task?
2. Is there a difference in familiar and novel tasks? Or is the rate the same?
3. How well does the new worker monitor, identify and self-correct errors?
4. What seems to have the most effect on the rate of work? (fear of failure, distraction, lack of interest or initiative, etc.)
5. Are there inappropriate behaviors?
6. What seems to provoke these behaviors?
7. What are the consequences of these behaviors?
8. How is communication helping or hurting on the job?
9. Are there adverse effects of attention, memory, organization, impulsiveness?
10. Are there stress reactions to amount or difficulty of work?

The speech-language pathologist can be instrumental in ensuring that the adolescent presents his/her own needs in light of the general skills for employment and the specific requirements for a particular job. They can do so through modeling, discussion of the need to balance old–new information with the listener in mind, and role playing using video taping. The adolescent can take turns playing the role of him/herself and the potential educator or employer. From these exercises and subsequent discussion, adolescents can emerge with a written set of guidelines accompanied by visual illustrations and/or specific examples for informing others about themselves and their needs. They can then test themselves with arranged practice interviews followed by discussion of critiques. The guidelines for explaining needs and accommodations vary according to different adolescents' personalities and communication skills, but suggestions are presented in Box 10–5.

BOX 10–5: *Guidelines for Presenting Myself and My Needs to Others*

1. Wait for the employer to ask about you and answer as specifically as you can.
2. Ask about the job before you begin telling more about yourself—ask then tell.
3. Explain your strengths first and then your most important needs for accommodations.
4. Explain the extra efforts you will make to prepare yourself before you discuss the accommodations you need from teachers or employers.
5. Be direct and adult in your requests for accommodations rather than overly demanding or "pathetic."

Altering Communication on the Job

Accommodations needed at the workplace often include altering the communication especially for giving and following directions. Even adolescents with mild special needs can misinterpret directions. Prospective employees with language processing difficulties can misunderstand the language in directions without the ability to clarify easily or in a timely manner; can misunderstand directions without realizing it; might impulsively begin to follow the first direction without listening to the entire message; might not become alert quickly enough and then respond only to the last part of the directions. To avoid these mistakes, the at risk new employee needs to regularly restate oral directions to check understanding.

Employers need to realize that understanding directions is a critical step in doing any job and may require extra time to ensure accurate communication for those at risk for language and that simply asking if the direction is clear may not be sufficient. They need to know that it is more effective for new employees to explain directions in their own words than to repeat verbatim something they may not have understood. Alternative communication (assistive listening/speaking devices, interpreters, pictorial signs for nonreaders, etc.) may have to be provided in many cases along with modification of work environments and policies in response to a special need. (Lord-Larson & McKinley, 1995).

Employers may be more cooperative in providing these kinds of communication adjustments when they realize that they are effective for many situations for all employees. The old adage, "A picture is worth a thousand words" and the long history of active listening often promoted in business communication trainings can be discussed in relation to necessary accommodations.

Understanding Plans, Monitoring and Modifying as Needed

The potential employee needs to know what plan is being put in place and why, to appreciate that the plan needs to be monitored to find flaws that then need to be addressed quickly for modifications to ensure success in doing the job. Adolescents and young adults vary in their ability to monitor on their own. The old–new learning principle is important for appreciating just how overloaded they may be with new processes and information. However, they need to be guided in monitoring, whenever possible, so they can identify problems and know how to proceed (call a meeting with the appropriate helper, put into place steps already anticipated in the plan, etc.).

It seems important to allow for control by the adolescent when possible and this requires training. Asking for a device to be repaired, reporting that a guard on a machine is loose, noting when slower speech is required for best understanding are important responsibilities best managed by the employee but it can be hard to communicate to busy people who may not always seem available. Even adolescents without special needs can have difficulty confronting situations requiring negotiating or complaining on the job. Each of these kinds of situations requires understanding of what is needed, what the employer is required to do and knowing an appropriate way to ask. Gobble et al. (1987) suggest four steps in goal setting regarding just such situations: 1) the two collaborators establish a specific goal (asking others to speak more slowly); 2) they then identify factors that might interfere (embarrassment, fear of seeming rude); 3) they establish realistic objectives for reaching the goal (perhaps practicing with coworkers before asking supervisors to slow down); and finally, 4) the adolescent worker charts progress toward the established goals or, if progress is limited, initiates further problem solving.

Helping Those Who Cannot Advocate for Themselves on the Job

When adolescents or young adults are not able to advocate adequately for themselves, they should, at the very least, be fully informed of what others have noticed or changed in the plan for accommodation. Extended time with a job trainer seems the ideal opportunity to continue the kind of collaboration that we have been discussing in this book. The trainer and employee can work together to identify problems, make new plans when necessary, inform others of how the plans are working, and so forth. We hope, in this arrangement, the client can begin to understand and internalize what the job trainer does or, at least, be able to explain what is being done on his or her behalf.

Pragmatic language skills become paramount on the job and the youngster who has difficulty knowing how to be appropriate may need direct training of communication skills for informing without tattling, asking for help or presenting suggestions at the right time and from the right person, for conversing without interfering with ongoing work, and for managing free time appropriately. Anticipation of problems can be facilitated in discussions with the employer about actual situations that have occurred in the job under consideration and the problems that might emerge given the particular language problems of the employee. There was a man with very limited knowledge or word meanings, for instance, who reported many misunderstandings between himself and co-workers. He had difficulty generalizing from one situation to the next because of his concrete understandings, so plans needed to be discussed for dealing appropriately with these situations. Role playing the necessary communications using the very misunderstandings that had or might occur was essential in helping this man function more appropriately.

■□ TRANSLATING THE SHOULDER-TO-SHOULDER APPROACH TO WORK

Many adolescents need continuing collaboration to ensure effective problem solving in the work place. Job coaches have been helpful to employers and their new employees with special needs and, when available, may be the best collaborators during the transition from school to work. Checking the adolescent's understanding of work routines and rules, both explicit and implicit, are important just as it was at the beginning of a new year in school. The collaboration needs to include discussion of the job requirements in light of possible, specific difficulties based on the employee's self-knowledge. Many adolescents with special needs find it hard to think ahead and this is an important time to help them anticipate difficulties. It is a skill they need to learn—thinking of possibilities and devising alternative plans before problems occur. When the initial understandings are in place—knowing the routines, rules, possible problems and plans—then the new employee needs to devise a self-monitoring system for checking implementation of plans and/or noting problems, that is, to schedule times for self-assessment. Problem solving becomes the guiding principle here: identify the problem, make a plan, check the plan and make a new one if necessary, keep at it until the problem is solved. Adolescents or young adults need to discover when and how to solve problems on their own whenever possible instead of prematurely asking for help and, just as important, to recognize when they cannot solve a problem without help. They need to understand the chain of command when they ask for help and to understand how to ask. A paraphrase of Hymes' (1971) early definition of communicative competence is helpful for guiding adolescent employees in knowing when to speak within their workday and when not to speak; in knowing what to say, with whom they should discuss various topics, in what way they should communicate and how much to say. Adolescents or young adults with language and learning problems may talk too much and waste a supervisor's time for instance, or they may complain too often or to the wrong people about unimportant issues. They may introduce their grievances at the wrong times without noticing the body language of their listener which is signaling that the timing is wrong for this discussion. They may have the knowledge and work skill required but not the interpersonal communication ability for survival on the job. It has been helpful in collaborating with adolescent clients and those who work with them to arrange the WH words describing communicative competence across the top of a paper; to discuss various situations that have occurred and to simply check the columns under words that describe appropriate and inappropriate aspects of the client's communication (see Box 10–6). Job trainers can help youngsters with special language or learning needs adjust to work and they can be effective collaborators during the learning period. If the potential employee has been actively engaged in a shoulder-to-shoulder, problem solving based collaboration throughout his or her adolescent years, this experience should be helpful in the transition to work.

BOX 10–6: *Identifying Communication in Conflicts at Work*

Name_____

Date_____

Short description of the situation. Tell what happened first, next, next. Try to remember and to write what each person said or did.

   Place a *check or X* under the following words to show what you did well and what mistake you made in this situation using the following questions as a guide:

1. Did I talk at the right time?
2. Did I talk about the right topic?
3. Did I talk to the right person about this?
4. Did I explain in a clear, reasonable way?
5. Did I give enough (too much?) information?

When	What (topic)	To Whom	How	How Much

■□ SUMMARY

This chapter has suggested the importance of preparing students for transitions to post-secondary schooling or employment by ensuring their understanding of their own language and learning needs through periodic comprehension checks of their learning needs and plans. The importance of enlisting and checking for student investment in the planning has been stressed along with descriptions of various reasons why students may have opted out of IEP sessions throughout their high school years. The discussion of students' understanding the accommodations they need, and the responsibility of the school or job site to provide accommodations is significant to ensure compliance along with a clear understanding of the students' responsibilities in the process. Various accommodations have been listed and discussed with specific suggestions about the adult collaborator's role along with a description for making an initial study plan. The need for monitoring and adjusting plans is extremely important to ensure success when there are special needs. It appears through this discussion that whether adolescents go on for formal education or go directly to work, they need to understand what they need, how to make appropriate plans including modifications and accommodations, the importance of monitoring and revising plans, and how to express their needs to others. The shoulder-to-shoulder problem solving approach seems especially important for ensuring successful transitions for adolescents.

Epilogue

Our original concerns about Brent suggest that with a shoulder-to-shoulder approach, he can feel more in control of his own learning than he does now. He can have the chance to share his frustrations about poor performance in spite of hard work and be guided in expanding his understanding of learning to include more than memorizing isolated facts. With a problem solving focus, Brent can improve his learning in a systematic way and also discover the efficacy of problem solving in his social life and at work. Brent can become knowledgeable about himself as a learner with implications for what he needs to do for himself and about what accommodations he needs others to provide at school and at work. He can learn how to advocate for himself with teachers and employers when armed with self-knowledge and information about available assistance. Brent may retain his profile of strengths and weakness but with self-knowledge, new "tools" and appropriate support from others through a collaborative, shoulder-to-shoulder problem solving approach he can better realize his potential as a high school student, employee and functioning adult. Brent can learn to identify remaining problems ten years after high school that reflected what he had not learned originally or had forgotten. He can evaluate his current need to learn those facts or skills and proceed to problem solve in order to do so. Brent can profit from this approach.

References

Aaron, P. G., & Baker, C. (1991). *Reading disabilities in college and high school: Diagnosis and management.* Parkton, MD: York Press.

AGS. (1989). *Peabody Individual Achievement Test, revised.* Circle Pines, MN: American Guidance Service.

American College Testing. (1996). *The college assessment of academic progress.* Iowa City, IA: American College Testing.

Amori, B., Dalton, E. F., & Tighe, P. L. (1993). *IDEA reading and writing proficiency test.* Brea, CA: Ballard & Tighe.

Andrews, M., & Summers, A. (1988). *Voice therapy for adolescents.* Boston, MA: College Hill Press.

Aune, B., & Friehe, M. (1996). Transition to postsecondary education: Institutional and individual issues. *Topics in Language Disorders, 16*(3), 1–22.

Aylward, G. (1998). Review of the comprehensive test of nonverbal intelligence. In J. C. Impara, & B. S. Plake, (Eds.). *The thirteenth mental measurements yearbook.* (pp. 310–312.) Lincoln, NE: Buros Institute of Mental Measurements.

Bahr, C. M., Nelson, N. W., & Van Meter, A. (1996). The effects of text-based and graphics based software tools on planning and organizing stories. *Journal of Learning Disabilities, 2,* 355–370.

Bain, A., Bailet, L., & Moats, L. (1991). *Written language disorders: Theory into practice.* (pp. 65–98). Austin, TX: Pro-Ed.

Banks, J. A., Beyer, B. K, Contreras, G., Craven, J., Ladson-Billians, G., McFarland, M. A., & Parker, W. C. (1995). *United States and its neighbors.* New York: Macmillan/McGraw-Hill School Publishing Company.

Barkley, R. (1994). The assessment of attention in children. In G. Reid Lyon (Ed.), *Frames of reference for the assessment of learning disabilities: New views on measurement issues.* Baltimore, MD: Paul Brookes Publishing.

Barkley, R. (1998). *Attention-deficit hyperactivity disorder: a handbook of diagnosis and treatment,* (2nd ed) New York, NY: Guilford Press.

Bashir, A. S., Goldhammer, R. F., & Bigaj, S. J. (2000). Facilitating self-determination abilities in adults with LLD: Case study of a postsecondary student. *Topics in Language Disorders, 21*(1), 52–67.

Baucam, J., Cole, G., Denny, P., Hinckley, J., & Villemaire, J. (1993). *Teaching a study skills system that works!* Putney, VT: Landmark College, Inc.

Bauer, A., Lynch, E., & Murphy, E. S. (1993). "Who's in Charge Here?": Establishing the structure in a classroom of students with severe behavioral disorders. In A. Bauer (Ed.), *Children who challenge the system.* Norwood, N.J.: Ablex Publishing.

Bauer, W. R., & Tutonis, J. (1996). Management and advocacy. In M. Ylvisaker & E.M. Gobble (Eds.), *Community re-entry for head injured adults.* Boston: College-Hill.

Bauman, J. F. (1983). Children's ability to comprehend main ideas in content textbooks. *Reading World, 22,* 322–331.

Baxter, R., Cohen, S., & Ylvisaker, M. (1985). Comprehensive cognitive assessment. In M. Ylvisaker (Ed.), *Head injury rehabilitation: Children and adolescents.* pp. 247–274. San Diego, CA: College-Hill Press.

Benard, B. (1990). *The case for peers.* Portland, OR: Northwest Regional Educational Laboratory.

Bergman, M. (1987). Social grace or disgrace: Adolescent social skills and learning disability subtypes. *Reading, Writing and Learning Disabilities, 3,* 161–166.

Berninger, V., Hart, T., Abbot, R. K., & Karovsky, P. (1992). Diagnosing writing disabilities with and without IQ: A flexible, developmental perspective. *Learning Disabilities Quarterly, 15,* 103–118.

Bettelheim, B., & Zelan, K. (1982). *On learning to read: The child's fascination with meaning.* New York: Knopf.

Blachowisc, C. L. (1994). Problem-solving strategies for academic success. In G. P. Wallach & K. G. Butler (Eds.), Language learning disabilities in school-age children and adolescents. (pp. 304–322) New York: Merrill.

Blank, M., Marquis, M. A., & Klimovitch, M. O. (1994). *Directing school discourse.* Tucson, AZ: Communication Skillbuilders.

Blank, M., Marquis, M. A., & Klimovitch, M. O. (1995). *Directing early discourse.* Tucson, AZ: Communication Skillbuilders.

Blank, M., & White, S. J. (1992). A model for effective classroom discourse. Predicated topics with reduced verbal demands. *Australasian Journal of Special Education, 16,* 32–34.

Bliss, L. (1992). A comparison of tactful messages by children with and without langauge impairment. *Language, Speech and Hearing Services in Schools, 23,* 343–347.

Bloom, B. (1965). *Taxonomy of educational objective. Handbook I. Cognitive domain.* New York: David McKay.

Bloom, L. M., Hood, L., & Lightbown, P. (1974). Imitation in language development: If, when and why. *Cognitive Psychology, 6,* 380–420.

Bracken, B. A., & McCallum, R. S. (1998). *The universal nonverbal intelligence test-UNIT.* Itasca, IL: Riverside Publishing Company.

Bransford, J. D. (1993). Who ya gonna call? Thoughts about teaching problem solving. In P. Hallinger, K. Leithwood, and J. Murphy (Eds.), *Cognitive perspectives on educational leadership* (pp. 171–191). New York: Teachers College Press.

Bransford, J. D., & Stein, B. S. (1984). *The ideal problem solver: A guide for improving thinking learning and creativity.* New York: W.H. Freeman & Company.

Brossell, G., & Ash, B. H. (1984) . An experiment with the wording of essay topics. *College Composition and Communication, 35,* 423–425.

Brown, J., Fischco, V., & Hanna, G. (1993). *Nelson-Denny reading test* (Forms G and H). Itasca, IL: Riverside Publishing.

Brown, J., Hammill, D., & Wiederhold, L. (1995). *Test of reading comprehension* (3rd ed.) (TORC-3). Austin, TX: Pro-Ed.

Brown, L., Sherbenau, R., & Johnsen, S. (1997). *Test of nonverbal intelligence* (3rd ed.) (TONI-3). Austin, TX: Pro-Ed.

Brownell, R. (2000a). *Receptive one-word picture vocabulary test-2000*. Novato, CA: Academic Therapy.

Brownell, R. (2000b). *Expressive one-word picture vocabulary test-2000*. Novato, CA: Academic Therapy.

Butler, K. G., & Wallach, G. P. (1996). Keeping on track to the twenty-first century. In G. P. Wallach & K. G. Butler (Eds.), *Language learning disabilities in school-age children and adolescents: Some principles and applications*. New York: Merrill/Macmillan College Publishing.

Buzan, T. (1974). *Use both sides of your brain*. New York: E.P. Dutton.

Calkins, L. (1983). *Lessons from a child: On the teaching and learning of writing*. Portsmouth, NH: Heinemann.

Calkins, L. (1991). *Presentation to the TAWL organization*. University of Cincinnati.

Carr, E. M., & Ogle, D. M. (1987). A strategy for comprehension and summarization. *Journal of Reading, 30*, 626–631.

Carroll, J., & Sapon, S. (1959). *Modern language aptitude test (MLAT): Manual*, San Antonio, TX: The Psychological Corporation.

Catts, H. W., & Kamhi, A.G. (1999). *Language and reading disabilities*. Boston: Allyn & Bacon.

Cazden, C. B. (1988). *Classroom discourse: The language of teaching and learning*. Portsmouth, NH: Heinemann.

Chamot, A. (1981). Applications of second langauge acquisition research to the bilingual classroom. *Focus: National Clearinghouse for Bilingual Education, 8*, 1–6.

Cohen, S. (1986). Educational re-integration and programming for children with head injuries. *Journal of Head Trauma Rehabilitation, 1*.

Cohen, P. A., Kulik, J. A., & Kulik, C-L. C. (1982). Educational outcomes of peer tutoring: A meta-analysis of findings. *Americal Educational Research Journal, 19*(1), 237–248.

Cohen, M., & Riel, M. M. (1989). The effect of distance audiences on students' writing. *American Educational Research Journal, 26*, 143–159.

Coon, D. (1992). *Introduction to Psychology* (6th ed.). St. Paul, MN: West Publishing.

CTB. (1989). *Comprehensive test of basic skills* (4th ed. Level 17–18).

CTB Macmillan/McGraw Hill. (1993). *CTB writing assessment system*. Monterey, CA: Author.

Cummins, J. (1981). The entry and exit fallacy in bilingual education. *National Association for Bilingual Education Journal, 4*, 25–60.

Cummins, J. (1984). *Bilingualism and special education: Issues in assessment and pedagogy*. Clevedon, Avon, England: Multilingual Matters.

Daiute, C., & Morse, F. (1994). Access to knowledge and expression: Multimedia writing tools for students with diverse needs and strengths. *Journal of Special Education Technology, 12*, 221–256.

Daly, D. A. (1988). *The freedom of fluency: An inspiring program to promote fluency in adolescents and adults*. East Moline, IL: LinguiSystems, Inc.

D'Angelo, F. (1984). Nineteenth-century forms/models of discourse. *College Composition and Communication, 35*, 31–34.

Danzer, G. A., Klor de Alva, J. J., Wilson, L. E. & Woloch, N. (1998). *The Americans*. Evanston, IL: McDougal Ittell.

Delis, D., Kramer, J., Kaplan, E., & Ober, B. (1994, 2000). California Verbal Learning Test. Austin, TX: Harcourt Brace.

Denckla, M. B. (1994). Measurement of executive function. In G. Reid Lyon (Ed.), Frames of *reference for the assessment of learning disabilities: New views on measurement issues*. Baltimore: Paul Brookes Publishing.

Deshler, D., & Graham, S. (1980). Tape-recording educational materials for secondary handicapped students. *Teaching Exceptional Children, 13*, 52–54.

Donahue, M. L. (1994). Differences in classroom discourse styles. In D. Ripich & N. Creaghead (Eds.), *School Discourse* (2nd ed., pp. 229–262). San Diego, CA: Singular.

Donahue, M., & Bryan, T. (1984). Communication skills and peer relations of learning disabled adolescents. *Topics in Language Disorders, 4*(1), 10–21.

Downey, D. M., & Snyder, L. E. (2000). College students with LLD: The phonological core as risk for failure in foreign language classes. *Topics in Language Disorders, 21*(1), 82–92.

Downey, D. M., & Snyder, L. E. (2001). Curricular accommodations for college students with langauge learning disabilities. *Topics in Language Disorders, 21*(2), 55–67.

Dunn, L., & Dunn, L. (1997). *Peabody Picture Vocabulary Test-III* (4rd ed.). Circle Pines, MN: American Guidance Association.

Durrell, D. D., & Catterson, J. H. (1980). *Durrell analysis of reading difficulty* (3rd ed.). Yonkers-on-Hudson, NY: World Book.

Ehren, B. J. (1994). New directions for meeting the academic needs of adolescents with language learning disabilities. In G. P. Wallach & K. G. Butler (Eds.), *Language learning disabilities in school-age children and adolescents: Some principles and applications*. (pp. 393–417) New York: Merrill, an imprint of Macmillan College Publishing Company.

Elbow, P. (1973). *Writing without teachers*. New York: Oxford University Press.

Ellis, D. B. (1991). Becoming a master student (6th ed.). Rapid City, SD: College Survival, Inc.

Englert, C., & Raphael, T. (1988). Constructing well formed prose: Process structure and metacognitive knowledge. *Exceptional Children, 54*(6), 513–520.

ERB. (1997). *ERB Writing Assessment Program, level III*. New York: Educational Records Bureau.

ETS. (1991). *Educational Testing Service Test of Applied Literacy Skills for Adults*. Princeton, NJ: Educational Testing Service.

Farmer, S. S. & Nesbit, E. (2000). The Triune Assessment-Intervention Model (TAIM) for students with sensemaking and dynamic literacy deficits. *Topics in Language Disorders, 21*(1), 30–51.

Farmer, S., & Sanchez, L. E. (1998). Time management profile. In Farmer, S., & Sanchez, L. E. Time management problems: Sequelae to language-learning disorders. *Rocky Mountain Journal of Communication Disorders, 12*, 12–19.

Feeney, T. J. & Yluisahaer, M. (1995). Choice and routine: Antecedent behavioral interventions for adolescents with severe traumatic brain injury. *Journal of Head Trauma Rehabilitation, 10*(3), 67–86.

Fisher, H. B., & Logemann, J. A. (1971). *The Fisher-Logemann test of articulation competence*. Austin, TX: Pro-Ed.

Gallagher, T. M. (1993). Language skills and the development of social competence in school-age children. *Language, Speech and Hearing Services in Schools*, 24(4), 199–205.

Ganschow, L., Phillips, L., & Schneider, E. (2001). Closing the gap: Accommodating students with language learning disabilities in college. *Topics in Language Disorders*, 21(2): 17–37.

Gardner, H. (1983). *Frames of minds.* New York: Basic Books.

Gardner, H. (1991). *The unschooled mind: How children think and how schools should teach.* New York: Basic Books.

Gartner, A., & Rieseman, F. (1993). *Peer tutoring. Toward a new model* (ERIC Digest). Washington, DC: Clearinghouse on Teaching and Teacher Education. (ERIC Document Reproduction Service Number No. ED 362 506).

Gee, J. P. (1996). *Social linguistics and literacies* (2nd ed.). Briston, PA: Taylor & Francis, Inc.

German, D. (1990). *Test of adolescent/adult word finding.* Austin, TX: Pro-Ed.

Gillet, J. W., & Temple, C. (1986). *Understanding reading problems: Assessment and instruction* (2nd ed.). Boston, MA: Litltle, Brown & Co.

Gilliam, J. (1995). *Attention-deficit/hyperactivity disorder test (ADHDT).* Austin, TX: Pro-Ed.

Ginott, H. (1971). *Between parent and teenager.* New York: Avon.

Glasser, W. (1993a). *The quality school.* New York: Harper Perennial.

Glasser, W. (1993b). *The quality school teacher: A companion volume to the quality school.* New York: HarperPerennial, a division of Harper Collins.

Glaub, V. E., & Kamphaus, R. W. (1991). *The Stanford-Binet Intelligence Scale* (4th ed., nonverbal short form). Itasca, IL: Riverside Publishing Company.

Gobble, E. M., Henry, K., Pfahl, J. C. & Smith, G. J. (1987). Work adjustment services. In M. Ylvisaker & E. M. Gobble, (Eds.), *Community re—entry for head injured adults* (pp. 221–258). Boston: College-Hill.

Goldman, R., & Fristoe, M. (2000). *The Goldman-Fristoe test of articulation–Two.* Circle Pines, MN: AGS.

Goldman, R., Fristoe, M & Woodcock, C.W. (1970). *The Goldman-Fristoe-Woodcock Test of Auditory Discrimination.* Circle Pines, MN: AGS.

Goldman, R., Fristoe, M., & Woodcock, C. W. (1976). *The Goldman-Fristoe-Woodcock Auditory Skills Battery.* Circle Pines, MN: AGS.

Goldstein, A., & McGinnis, E. (1997). *Skillstreaming the Adolescent: New strategies and perspectives for teaching prosocial skills.* Champaign, IL: Research Press.

Goodlad, S., & Hirst, B. (1989). *Peer tutoring: A guide to learning by teaching.* New York: Nichols Publishing.

Goodman, Y., & Burke, C. (1972). *Reading miscue inventory: Procedure for diagnosis and evaluation.* New York: The Macmillian Company.

Gordon, T. (1976). *PET in action.* New York: Wyden.

Gould, B. (1991). Curricular strategies for written expression. In A. Bain, L. Bailet, & L. Moats (Eds.) *Written language disorders: Theory into practice* (pp. 129–164). Austin, TX: Pro-Ed.

Gragg, C. (1940). Because wisdom can't be told. *Harvard Alumni Bulletin*, Reprinted Harvard Business School, # 451–005.

Grandin, T. (1995). *Thinking in pictures: And other reports from my life with autism.* New York: Vintage Books.

Graves, D. (1983). *Writing: Teachers and children at work.* Exeter, NH: Heinemann.

Graves, D. (1985). *Teaching writing.* Writer in Residence Lecture. Miami University, Oxford, OH.

Greenberg, K. (1981). *The effects of variations in essay questions on the writing per-formance of CUNY freshman.* New York: The City University of New York Instructional Resource Center.

Greenwood, C. R., Delquadri, J. C., & Hall, R. V. (1989). Longitudinal effects of classwide peer tutoring. *Journal of Educational Psychology, 81*(3) 371–383.

Grice, H. (1975). Logic and conversation. In P. Cole & J. Morgan (Eds.), *Syntax and semantics: Speech acts* (Vol. 3) (pp. 41–58). New York: Academic Press.

Hammill, D. D. & Bryant, B. R. (1991). *Detroit Tests of Learning Aptitude–Adult.* Austin:TX, Pro-Ed.

Hammill, D., Brown, V. Larsen, S., & Wiederholt, J. L. (1994). *Test of Adolescent and Adult Language,* (3rd ed.). Austin, TX: Pro-Ed.

Hammill, D., & Larsen, S. (1996). *Test of written language* (3rd ed.). Austin, TX: Pro-Ed.

Hammill, D. D., Pearson, N. A., & Wiederholt, L. J. (1996). *Comprehensive test of nonverbal intelligence.* Austin, TX: Pro-Ed.

Harcourt Brace Educational Measurement of the Psychological Corporation. (1991). *The Stanford writing assessment program,* (2nd ed.). San Antonio, TX: Author.

Harcourt Brace (1992a). *Stanford achievement tests: Listening Comprehension test.* Austin, TX: Harcourt Brace Educational Measurements.

Harcourt Brace. (1992b). *Metropolitan Achievement Tests* (7th ed.), Austin, TX: Harcourt Brace Educational Measurements.

Harris, T. (1969). *I'm ok—you're ok.* New York and Evanston: Harper & Row.

Harvey, S., & Goudis, A. (2000). *Strategies that work: Teaching comprehension to enhance understanding,* York, ME: Stenhouse Publishers.

Health Resource Center (1992). *Transition resource guide.* Washington, DC: Author.

Heaton, R. K., Chehine, G. J., Talley, J. L., Hay, G. G., & Curtiss, G. (1981–1993). *The Wisconsin card sort test.* Odessa, FL: Psychological Assessment Resources.

Heden, D. (1987). Students as teachers: A tool for improving school climate and productivity. *Social Policy, 17*(3), 42–47.

Hess, A. (1998). Review of the Wechsler adult intelligence scale, (3rd ed.). In J. C. Impara, & B. S. Plake (Eds.), *The thirteenth mental measurements yearbook.* (pp. 345–348). Lincoln, NE: Buros Institute of Mental Measurements.

Highnam, C. L. (1994). Cognition. In W. O. Haynes, & B. B. Shulman (Eds.), *Communication development: Foundations, processes and clinical applications.* (pp. 114–134). Englewood Cliffs, NJ: Prentice Hall.

Hirsch, E. D., Jr. (1987). *Cultural literacy: What every American needs to know.* Boston: Houghton-Mifflin.

Hoetker, J., & Brossell, G. (1989). The effects of systematic variations in essay topics on the writing performance of college freshman. *College Composition and Communication, 40,* 414–421.

Hooper, S. R., Montgomer, J., Swartz, C., Reed, M. S., Sandler, S. D., Levine, M. D. Watson, T. E., & Wasileski, T. (1994). Measurement of written language expression. In G. Reid Lyon (Ed.) *Frames of reference for the assessment of learn-ing disabilities: New views on measurement issues* (pp. 375–418). Baltimore, MD: Paul Brookes Publishing.

Howie, S. H. (1984). *A guide for teaching writing in content areas.* Boston: Allyn & Bacon.

Hymes, D. (1971). Competence and performance in linguistic theory. In R. Huxley & E. Ingram (Eds.), *Language acquisition: Models and methods.* New York: Academic Press.

Jennett, B., & Teasdale, G., (1981). *Management of head injuries.* Philadelphia: F. A. Davis.

Johns, J. (1997). *Basic reading inventory: Pre-primer through Grades 12 and early literacy assessments* (7th ed.). Dubuque, IA: Kendall/Hunt Publishing.

Johnson, D. & Pearson, P. (1984). *Teaching reading comprehension* (2nd ed.). New York: Holt, Rinehart & Winston.

Johnson, K. L., & Heinze, B. A. (1994). *The fluency companion: Strategies for stuttering intervention.* East Moline, IL: LinguiSystems.

Johnston, J. R. (1982). Interpreting the Leiter IQ: Performance profiles of young and normal and language-disordered children. *Journal of Speech and Hearing Research, 25,* 291–296.

Kahmi, A. G., Minor, J. S., & Mauer, D. (1990). Content analysis and intratest performance profiles on the Columbia and the TONI. *Journal of Speech and Hearing Research, 33,* 375–379.

Kamphaus, R. W. (1995). Review of the SIT-R. In J. C. Conoley, & J. C. Impara, (Eds.) *The twelfth mental measurements yearbook* (pp. 954–956). Lincoln, NB: Buros Institute of Mental Measurements.

Karlsen, G. & Gardner, E. (1995). Stanford Diagnostic Reading Test, (4th ed.) (SKRT4). San Antonio, TX: Harcourt Brace Educational Measurments.

Kaufman, A. S. (1979). *Intelligent testing with the WISC-R.* New York: Wiley.

Kaufman, A., & Kaufman, N. (1985, renormed in 1997). *Kaufman Test for Educational Achievement, comprehensive form.* Circle Pines, MN: American Guidance Service.

Kaufman, A. S., & Kaufman, N. L. (1990). *K-BIT: The Kaufman brief intelligence test.* Circle Pines, MN: AGS.

Kaufman, A. S., & Kaufman, N. L. (1993). *The Kaufman adolescent and adult intelligence test.* Circle Pines, MN: AGS.

Keith, R. W. (1994). *SCAN-A: A test for auditory processing disorders in adolescents and adults.* San Antonio, TX: Psychological Corporation.

Kimmel, E. W. (1998). Review of the Writing Process Test. In J. C. Impara, & B. S. Plake, (Eds.), *The thirteenth mental measurements yearbook* (pp. 1159–1161). Lincoln, NE: Buros Institute of Mental Measurements.

Klein, M. (1985). *The development of writing in children: Pre-K through grade 8.* Englewood Cliffs, NJ: Prentice-Hall.

Kriegel, R., & Patler, L. (1991). *If it ain't broke ... break it!* New York: Time Warner Books.

Langer, E. J. (1989). *Mindfulness.* Reading, MS: Addison-Wesley.

Langer, J. A. (1981). From theory to practice: A prereading plan. *Journal of Reading, 25,* 152–156.

Larsen, S. C., Hammill, D. D., & Moats, L. (1999). *Test of written spelling* (4th ed.). Austin, TX: Pro-Ed.

Lenz, B. K., Bulgren, J., & Hudson, P. (1990). Content enhancement: A model for promoting the acquisition of content by individuals with learning disabilities. In E. E. Scruggs & B. L.Wong (Eds.), *Intervention research in learning disabilities* (pp. 122–165). New York: Springer-Verlag.

Levine, M. (1990). *Intention, attention, retention.* Presentation to the Attention Deficit Disorder Parent Support Group. Cincinnati, OH.

Lewis, J., & Greene, J. (1982). *Thinking better.* New York: Rawson, Wade Publishers, Inc.

Lindamood, C., & Lindamood, P. (1979). *Lindamood auditory conceptualization test*. Austin, TX: Pro-Ed.

Lindamood, P. C. (1994). Issues in researching the link between phonological awareness, learning disabilities and spelling. In G. R. Lyon (Ed.), *Frames of reference for the measurement of learning disabilities: New views on measurement issues* (pp. 351–374). Baltimore, MD: Paul Brookes Pub. Co.

Lindfors, J. (1980). *Children's language and learning*. Englewood Cliffs, NJ: Prentice-Hall.

London, R. (1993). *A curriculum of nonroutine problems*. AERA Convention.

Lord-Larson, V., & McKinley, N. (1995). *Language disorders in older students: Preadolescents and adolescent*. Eau Claire, WIO: Thinking Publications.

Lounsbury, J., & Clark, D. (1990). *Inside grade eight: From apathy to excitement*. Reston, VA: National Association of Secondary School Principals.

Lounsbury, J., & Johnston, J. (1985). *How fares the ninth grade? A day in the life of a 9th grader*. Reston, VA: National Association of Secondary School Principals.

Lounsbury, J., & Johnston, J. (1988). *Life in three sixth grades*. Reston, VA: National Association of Secondary School Principals.

Luetke-Stahlman, B. (1998). The Cummins model and applications. In B. Luetke-Stahlman (Ed.) *Language issues in deaf education* (pp. 63–85). Hillsboro, OR: Butte Publishing.

Lundsteen, S. (1974). Questioning to develop creative problem solving. *Elementary English, 51*(5), 645–660.

Macarthur, C. A., (2000). New tools for writing assistance technology for students with writing difficulties. *Topics in Language Disorders, 20*(4), 85–100.

Maginitie, W. H., & Maginitie, R. K. (1989). *Gates-Maginitie Reading Tests* (3rd ed.). Itasca, IL: Riverside Publishing.

Manzo, A. V. (1969). The ReQuest procedure. *Journal of Reading, 11*, 123–125.

Marston, D. B. (1989). A curriculum-based measurement approach to assessing academic performance: What is is and why do it. In M.R. Shinn (Ed.), *Curriculum-based measurement: Assessing special children* (pp.18–78). New York: Guilford Press.

McCauley, R. J., & Swisher, L. (1984). Psychometric review of language and articulation tests for preschool children. *Journal of Speech & Hearing Disorders, 49* 34–42.

McKechnie, J .L. (1983). *Webster's new twentieth centeury dictionary of the English language, unabridged*. New York: Simon and Schuster.

Merritt, D. D., Barton, J., & Culatta, B. (1998). Instructional discourse: A framework for learning. In D. D. Merritt & B. Culatta, (Eds.), *Language Intervention in the classroom* (pp. 143–174). San Diego, CA: Singular Publishing.

Merritt, D. D., & Culatta, B. (1998). *Language Intervention in the classroom*. San Diego, CA: Singular Publishing.

Meyers, J. E., & Meyers, K. R. (1995). *Rey complex figure test and recognition trial*. Odessa, FL: Psychological Assessment Resources.

Miller, G., & Gildea, P. (1987). How children learn words. *Scientific American, 257*, 94–99.

Miller, L. (1990). *The smart profile: A qualitative approach for describing learners and designing instruction*. Austin, TX: Smart Alternatives.

Miller, L. (1993). *What we call smart: A new narrative for intelligence and learning*. San Diego, CA: Singular Publishing Group.

Miller, L. (1994). *The QuickSMART profile*. Austin, TX: Smart Alternatives.

Moats, L. (1994). Assessment of spelling in learning disabilities research. In G. Reid Lyon (Ed.) *Frames of reference for the assessment of learning disabilities; New views on measurement issues* (pp.333– 350). Baltimore, MD: Paul Brookes Publishing.

Moffett, J. (1986). *Teaching the universe of discourse.* Boston: Houghton-Mifflin.

Morgan, D. L., & Guilford, A. M. (1984). *The adolescent language screening test.* Austin, TX: Pro-Ed.

Morine-Dershimer, G. (1985). *Talking, listening and learning in elementary school classrooms.* New York: Longman.

Muma, J. (1978). *Language handbook: Concepts, assessment, intervention.* Englewood Cliffs, NJ: Prentice-Hall.

Murray-Ward, M. (1998). Review of Nelson-Denny test of reading. In J. C. Impara, & B. S. Plake (Eds.), *The thirteenth mental measurements yearbook.* Lincoln, NE: Buros Institute of Mental Measurements.

Nelson, N. (1989). Curriculum-based language assessment and intervention. *Language, Speech, and Hearing Services in Schools, 20,* 170–184.

Nelson, N. (1994). Curriculum-based language assessment and intervention across the grades In G. P. Wallach & K. G. Butler (Eds.), *Language learning disabilities in school—age children and adolescents: Some principles and applications* (pp. 104–131). New York: Merrill, an imprint of Macmillan College Publishing.

Nelson, N. (1998). *Childhood language disorders in context: Infancy through adolescence.* (2nd ed.). Boston:MA: Allyn & Bacon.

Newman, A. P., Lewis, W., & Beverstock, C. (1993). *Prison literacy.* Philadelphia: National Center on Adult Literacy.

Nicholson, C. Slosson Oral Reading Test, 1990.

Nippold, M. (1988). *Later language development: Ages 9 through 19.* Boston: College-Hill.

O'Connor, J. R. & Goldberg, R. M. (1980). *Exploring American citizenship.* New York: Globe Book Company.

Ogle, D. (1986). K-W-L: A teaching model that develops active reading of expository text. *The Reading Teacher, 39*(6), 564–570.

Palinscar, A. S. (1986). Metagcognitive strategy instruction. *Exceptional Children. 53*(2), 118–24.

Palincsar, A. S., & Brown, A. L. (1984). Reciprocal teaching of comprehension fostering and comprehension monitoring activities. *Cognition and Instruction, 1*(1), 117–175.

Paton, J. W. (2001). Living and working with a central auditory processing disorder (CAPD). *LD on Line.* Retrieved May 5, 2001 from the World Wide Web: *Http///www.ldonline.orglld_indepth/process_deficit/living_working. html*

Paul, M. (1991). *When words are bars.* Kitchener, Ontario: Core Literacy.

Pearson, P. D., & Johnson, D.D. (1978). *Teaching reading comprehension.* New York: Holt, Rinehart & Winston.

Perera, K. (1986). Some linguistic difficulties in school textbooks. In B. Gillham (Ed.), *The language of school subjects* (pp. 53–67). London: Heinemann Educational Books.

Perkins, D. (1992). *Smart schools: From training memories to educating minds.* New York: The Free Press, Division of MacMillan.

Perrin, L. (Ed.). (1986). *Understanding psychology* (4th ed.). New York: Random House.

Prendeville, J. (1991). *A study of two preschool children's narrating abilities in spontaneous conversation.* Unpublished dissertation. University of Cincinnati.

Prigatano, G. P. et al. (1986). *Neuropsychological rehabilittion after brain injury.* Baltimore: Johns Hopkins University Press.

Putallaz, M., & Gottman, J. (1981). An interactional model of children's entry into peer groups. *Child Development, 52,* 986–994.

Resnick, L. B. (1987). Learning in school and out. *Educational Researcher, 16*(9), 13–20.

Reynolds, C. R., & Bigler, E. D. (1994). *The test of memory and learning.* Austin, TX: Pro-Ed.

Richards, R. (1998). Review of the educational testing service test of applied literacy skills for adults In J. C. Impara & B.S. Plake (Eds.), *The thirteenth mental measurements yearbook* (pp. 429–431). Lincoln, NE: Buros Institute of Mental Measurements.

Robinson, F. (1962). *Effective reading.* New York: Harper and Brothers.

Robinson, H. A. (1978). *Teaching reading and study skills: The content areas* (2nd ed.). Boston: Allyn & Bacon.

Rogers, B. (1998). Review of the Wechsler adult intelligence scale (3rd ed.). In J. C. Impara & B. S. Plake, (Eds.), *The thirteenth mental measurements yearbook* (pp. 348–352). Lincoln, NE: Buros Institute of Mental Measurements.

Rogers, C. (1942). *Counseling and psychotherapy.* Cambridge, MA: Houghton-Mifflin.

Roid, G. H., & Miller, L. (1996). *The Leiter-R.* Chicago: Stoelting Company.

Ross-Swain, D. (1996). *Ross Information Processing Assessment* (2nd ed.). Austin, TX: Pro-Ed.

Rourke, B.P. (1994). Neuropsychological assessment of children with learning disabilities: Measurement issues. In G.R. Lyons (Ed.). *Frames of reference for the assessment of learning disabilities: New views on measurement issues.* (pp. 475–514) Baltimore, MD: Paul H. Brookes Publishing Co.

Rourke, B. P., & Adams, K. M. (1984). Quantitative approach to the neuropsychologica assessment of children. In R. E. Tarter & G. Goldstein (Eds.), *Advances in clinical neuropsychology, (Vol. 2,* pp. 79–108). New York; Plenum.

Rourke, B. P., Baker, D. J., Fisk, J. L. & Strang, J. D. (1983). *Child neuropsychology: An introduction to theory, research, and clinical practice.* New York: Guilford Press.

Rourke, B. P., Fisk, J. L. & Strang, J. D. (1986). *Neuropsychological assessment of children: A treatment oriented approach.* New York: Guilford Press.

Salomon, G. (1992). *Metagognitive facilitation and cultivation during essay writing: The case of the Writing Partner.* Paper presented at the Third Internal Conference on Cognitive Education. Riverside, CA.

Salvia, J., & Ysseldyke, J. E. (1991). *Assessment in special and remedial education* (5th ed.). Boston: Houghton Mifflin Company.

Schaeffer, A. L., Zigmond, N., Kerr, M. M., & Farra, H. E. (1990). Helping teenagers develop school survival skills. *Teaching Exceptional Children, 23*(1), 6–9.

Schneider, E., Philips, L. & Ganschow, L. (2000, July). *Mind the gap: Student and professor perspectives on learning in foreign language substitution classes.* Presentation at the International Academy for Research in Learning Disabilities (IARLD), Vancouver, BC, Canada.

Schretian, D. (1997). *Brief test of attention.* Odessa, FL: Psychological Assessment Resources.

Schumaker, J. B.. & Hazel, J. S. (1984). Social skills assessment and training for the learning disabled: Who's on first what's on second? Part II. *Journal of Learning Disabilities, 17,* 492–499.

Schwartz, S. H., & Perkins, D. N. (1994). Teaching the metacurriculum: A new approach to enhancing subject learning. In D. N. Perkins, J. L. Schwartz, M. M. West, & M. S. Wiske (Eds.), *Software goes to school: Teaching for understanding in the age of technology* (pp. 255–270). New York: Oxford University Press.

Semel, E., Wiig, E. H., & Secord, W. A. (1994). *Clinical evaluation of language fundamentals,* (3rd ed.). San Antonio: The Psychological Corporation.

Shames, G., & Florance, C. (1980). *Stutter-free speech.* Columbus, OH: Charles E. Merrill.

Shinn, M. R. (Ed.). (1989). *Curriculum-based measurement: Assessing special children.* New York: Guilford Press.

Siegel, L., (1992). An evaluation of the discrepancy definition of dyslexia. *Journal of Learning Disabilities,* 25, 618–629.

Simon, C. (1986). Evaluating communicative competence (Rev. ed.). Tucson, AZ: Communication Skill Builders.

Simon, C. (1991). *The communication questionnaire.* Personal correspondence.

Simon, J. A. (2001). Legal issues in serving postsecondary students with disabilities. *Topics in Language Disorders,* 21(2), 1–16.

Slosson, R. Nicholson, C. L. & Hibpshman, T. H. (1991). *The Slosson intelligence test* (revised). East Aurora, NY: Slosson Educational Publishing, Inc.

Smith, F. (1988). *Joining the literacy club: Further essays into education.* Portsmouth, NH: Heinemann.

Smith, P. K. (1998). *Review of Nelson-Denny reading test* (Forms G and H). In J. C. Impara, & B. S. Plake, (Eds.), *The thirteenth mental measurements yearbook* (pp. 685–686). Lincoln, NE: Buros Institute of Mental Measurements.

Spache, G. (1995). *Diagnostic reading scales.* Monterey, CA: California Test Bureau, McGraw Hill.

Stauffer, R. G. (1969). *Directing reading maturity as a cognitive process.* New York: Harper & Row.

Stauffer, R. G., & Cramer, R. (1968) *Teaching critical reading at the primary level.* Newark, NJ: Del International Reading Association.

Sternberg, R. J. (1981). The nature of intelligence. *New York University Education Quarterly,* 12, 10–17.

Strichart, S. S., & Mangrum II, C. T. (1993). *Teaching study strategies to students with learning disabilities.* Boston, MS: Allyn & Bacon.

Swengel, E. M. (1991). Peer tutoring: Back to the roots of peer helping. *The Peer Facilitator Quarterly,* 8(4), 28–32).

Szekeres, S. F., Ylvisaker, M. & Cohen, S. B. (1987). A framework for cognitive rehabilitation therapy. In M. Ylvisaker & E. M. Gobble (Eds.), *Community reentry for head Injury* (pp. 87–136). Boston: MA: College-Hill/Litt, Brown & Company.

Tallal, P. (1980). Auditory temporal processing, phonics and reading disablities in children. *Brain and Language,* 9, 182–198.

Tallal, P., Miller, S. I., Bedi, G., Byma, G., Wang, X., Nagarajan, S. S., Schriener, C., Jenkins, W. M., & Merzenich, M. M. (1996). Language comprehension in language-learning impaired children improved with acoustically modified speech. *Science,* 271, 81–84.

Tallal, P., & Percy, M. (1978). Defects of auditory perception in children with developmental dysphasia. In A. Wlyke (Ed.), *Developmental dysphasia* (pp. 63–84). New York: Academic Press.

Tallal, P., & Stark, R. (1976). Relation between speech perception and speech production impairment in children with developmental dysphasia. *Brain and Language,* 3, 305–317.

Tattershall, S. (1994a). Shoulder-to-shoulder: Collaborating with adolescents regarding discourse strategies. In D. Ripich & N. Creaghead (Eds.), *School Discourse,* (2nd ed., pp. 43–372). San Diego,CA: Singular.

Tattershall, S. (1994b). Upping the ante: Increasing demands for literacy and discourse skills. In D. Ripich & N. Creaghead (Eds.), *School Discourse,* (2nd ed., pp. 63–90). San Diego, CA: Singular.

Tattershall, S., & Prendeville, J. (1993). *Questions and Answers.* ASHA, Washington, DC presentation.

Thorum, A.R. 1986).*The Fullerton language test for adolescents,* (2nd ed.) . Austin, TX: Pro-Ed.

Tonjes, M. (1986). Reading and thinking skills required in the subject classroom. In B. Gillham (Ed.), *The Language of school subjects* (pp. 68–75). London: Heinemann Educational Books.

Tucker, J. A. (1985). Curriculum—based assessment: An introduction. *Exceptional Children, 52,* 199–204.

Van Allsburg, C. (1984). *The mysteries of Harris Burdick.* Boston: Houghton-Mifflin.

van Dijk, T. A. (1980). *Macrostructure.* Hillsdale, NJ: Lawrence Erlbaum Associates.

van Kleek, A. (1994). Metalinguistic development. In G. P. Wallach & K. G. Butler, (Eds.), *Language learning disabilities in school-age children and adolescents: Some principles and applications* (pp. 53–98). New York: Merrill, an imprint of Macmillan College Publishing.

Vellutino, F. (1979b). The validity of the perceptual deficit explanation of reading disability. A reply to Fletcher and Saby. *Journal of Learning Disabilities, 12,* 27–34.

Viise, N. M. (1992). *A comparison of child and adult spelling development.* Unpublished doctoral disssertation. University of Virginia.

Vygotsky, L. S. (1978). *Mind in society: The development of higher psychological processes.* Cambridge, MA: Harvard University Press.

Wachter, J. F., Fawber, H. L., & Scott, M. B. (1987). Treatment aspects of vocational evaluation and placement for traumatically brain injured adults. In M. Ylvisaker & E. M. Gobble, (Eds.), *Community re-entry for head injured adults* (pp. 259–300). Boston: College-Hill.

Wagner, R., Torgesen, J., & Rashotte, C. (1999). *Comprehensive test of phonological processing.* Austin, TX: Pro-Ed.

Wagner, R. K. (1993). Practical problem-solving. In P. Hallinger, K. Leithwood, & J. Murphy, (Eds.), *Cognitive perspectives on educational leadership.* (pp. 88–102). New York: Teachers College Press.

Wallace, G., & Hamill, D.D. (1994). *The comprehensive receptive and expressive vocabulary test.* Austin, TX: Pro-Ed.

Wallace, G., & Hamill, D. D. (1997). *The comprehensive receptive and expressive vocabulary test-adult and the computer administered version.* Austin, TX: Pro-Ed.

Wallace, M. (1982). *Teaching vocabulary.* London: Heinemann Educational Books.

Wallach, G. P., & Butler, K. G. (1994). *Language learning disabilities in school-age children and adolescents: Some principles and applications.* New York: Merrill, an imprint of Macmillan College Publishing.

Wallach, G., & Miller, L. (1988). *Language intervention and academic success.* Austin, TX: Pro-Ed.

Warden, M. R., & Hutchinson, T. K. (1992). *Writing Process Test (WPT).* Itasca, IL: Riverside Publishing.

Weaver, C. (1980). *Psycholinguistics and reading: From process to practice.* Cambridge, MA: Winthrop.

Weaver, C. (1994) *Reading process and practice: From socio—linguistics to whole language* (2nd ed.). Portsmouth, NH: Heinemann.

Wechsler, D. (1939–1997a). *Wechsler intelligence scale for children* (3rd ed.). Austin, TX: Pro Ed.

Wechsler, D. (1939–1997b). *Wechsler adult intelligence scale* (3rd ed.). Austin, TX: Pro Ed.

Weinstein, C., & Palmer, D. (1990). *Learning and Study Strategies-High School (LASSI-HS).* Clearwater, FL: H & H Publishing.

Weinstein, C., & Palmer, D., & Schulte, A. (1987). *Learning and Study Strategies-High School (LASSI).* Clearwater, FL: H & H Publishing.

Weiss, C. E. (1980). *The Weiss comprehensive articulation test.* Austin, TX: Pro-Ed.

Wells, G. (1999). *Dialogic inquiry: Towards a sociocultural practice and theory of education.* New York: Cambridge University Press.

Wertime, R. (1979). Students problems and courage spans. In J. Lockhead & J. Clements (Eds.), *Cognitive process instruction.* Philadelphia: The Franklin Institute Press.

Westby, C. (1985). Learning to talk—Talking to learn: Oral—literate language differences. In C. Simon (Ed.), *Communication skills and classroom success: Therapy methodologies for language learning disabled students.* (pp. 181–213) San Diego, CA: College-Hill Press.

Westby, C., & Costlow, L. (1991). Implementing a whole language program in a special education class. *Topics in Language Disorders, 1*(3), 69–84.

Whaley, J. (1981). Story grammars and reading instruction. *The Reading Teacher, 34*(8), 762–771.

Whimbey, A., & Lockhead, R. (1982). *Problem solving and comprehension.* Philadelphia: Franklin Institute Press.

Whitmire, K. A. (2000). Adolescence as a developmental phase: A tutorial. *Topics in Language Disorders, 20*(2), 1–14.

Wiederhold, C. (1997). *The q-matrix/cooperative learning & higher-level thinking.* San Clemente, CA: Kagan Cooperative Learning.

Wiederholt, J. L., & Blalock, G. (2000). *Gray silent reading tests.* Austin, TX: Pro-Ed.

Wiederholt, J. L., & Bryant, B.R (1992). *The Gray oral reading test—GORT-3.* Austin, TX. Pro-Ed.

Wiig, E. H., & Secord, W. (1989). *Test of language competenc— Expanded Edition.* San Antonio: TX: The Psychological Corporation.

Wilkinson, G. S. (1994). *The wide range achievement test,* (3rd ed.). Austin, TX: Pro-Ed.

Williams, J. (1985). How to teach readers to find the main idea. In F. L. Harris & E. J. Cooper (Eds.), *Reading, thinking and concept development,* New York: College Entrance Examination Board. pp. 21–32.

Williams, K. T. (1997). *Expressive vocabulary test.* Circle Pines, MN: AGS.

Wong, B., & Wong, R. (1988). Cognitive interventions for learning disabilities. In K.Kavale (Ed.). Learning Disabilities: State of the art and practice. Boston, MA: Little Brown.

Wood, K. (1984). Probable passage: a writing strategy. *The Reading Teacher, 37*(6), 496–499.

Woodcock, R. (1987). *Woodcock reading mastery tests* (revised, NU). Circle Pines, MN: American Guidance Service.

Woodcock, R. (1999). Woodcock Reading Mastery Tests-Revised, NV. Circle Pines, MN: American Guidance Service.

Woodcock, R. W., & Johnson, W. B. (1990). *Woodcock-Johnson Psychoeducational Battery-revised-Tests of Achievement, Standard Battery and Supplemental Battery.* Itasca, IL: Riverside Publishing.

Ylvisaker, M., & DeBonis, D. (2000). Executive function impairment in adolescence: TBI and ADHD. *Topics in Language Disorders, 20*(2), 29–55.

Ylvisaker, M., Feeney, J., & Feeney, T. (1999). An everyday approach to long-term rehabilitation after traumatic brain injury. In B. Cornet (Ed.), *Clinical practice management in speech-languagepathology: Principles and practicalities* (pp. 117–162). Gaithersburg, MD: Aspen Publishers.

Zachman, L., Huisingh, R., Barrett, M., Orman, J., & Blagden, C. (1989). *The word test: Adolescent.* Moline, IL: Lingui-Systems.

Bibliography

Bar-on, R. (1997). *Bar-On emotional quotient inventory.* North Tonawand, NY: Multi-Health Systems, Inc.

Bennett-Kastor, T. L. (1986). Cohesion and predication in child narrative. *Journal of Child Language, 13,* 353–370.

Brinckerhoff, L. C., Shaw, S. F., & McGuire, J. M. (1992). Promoting access, accommodations and independence for college students with learning disabilities. *Journal of Learning Disabilities, 25,* 417–429.

Brown, A. L., & Palincsar, A. S. (1989). Guided cooperative learning and individual knowledge acquisition. In L. Resnick (Ed.), *Knowing, learning and instruction: Essays in honor of Robert Glaser.* Hillsdale, NJ: Lawrence Erbaum.

Brown, J. I., Bennett, J. M., & Hanna, G. (1981). *Nelson-Denny reading test.* Itasca, IL: Riverside Publishing Company.

Bryant, B. R., & Wiederholt, J. L. (1991). *The Gray oral reading test–diagnostic.* Austin, TX: Pro-Ed.

Crewe, N., & Athelstan, G. (1981). Functional assessment in vocational rehabilitation: A systematic approach to diagnosis and goal setting. *Archives of Physical Medicine and Rehabilitation, 62*(7), 299–305.

Crewe, N., & Athelstan, G. (1984). *Functional assessment inventory manual.* Menomonie, WI: Materials Development Center, Stout Vocational Rehabilitation Institute.

Cummins, J. (1986). Empowering minority students: A framework for intervention. *Harvard Educational Review, 56*(1), 18–36.

Damico, J. S. (1990). Prescriptionism as a motivating mechanism: An ethnographic study in the public schools. *Journal of Childhood Communication Disorders, 13,* 85–92.

Davidson, J. L., & Wilkerson, B. C. (1988). *Directed reading thinking activities.* Monroe, NY: Trillium Press.

Destafano, J. S., & Kantor, R. (1988). Cohesion in spoken and written dialogue: An investigation of cultural and textual constraints. *Linguistics and Education, 1,* 105–124.

Dunn R., & Griggs, S. A. (1995). *Multiculturalism and learning style*. Westport, CT: Praeger Publishing.

Farmer, S. (1995). *Test complexity index: Unpublished clinical material*. Las Cruces, NM: New Mexico State University.

Fey, M. E. (1986). *Language intervention with young children*. Needham, MA: Allyn & Bacon.

Flores d'Arcais, G. B. (1978). Levels of semantic knowledge in children's use of connectives. In A. Sinclair, R. J. Jarvella, & W. J. M. Levels (Eds.), *The child's conception of language* (pp. 133–155). New York: Springer-Verlag.

Flynt, E. S., & Cooter, R. B. (1995). *The Flynt-Cooter reading inventory* (2nd ed.). Scottsdale, AZ: Gorsuch Scarisbrick Publishers.

Gartner, A. (1992). *A peer-centered school*. New York: Peer Research Laboratory.

Gregg. N. (1985). College learning disabled, normal and basic writers: A comparison of frequency and accuracy of cohesive ties. *Journal of Psychoeducational Assessment, 3*, 223–231.

Gregg, N. (1991). Disorders of written expression. (In A. Bain, L. Bailet, & L. Moats, (Eds.) *Written language disorders: Theory into practice* (pp. 65–98). Austin, TX: Pro-Ed.

Gregg, N., & Hoy, C. (1990). Identifying the learning disabled. *Journal of College Admissions, 129*, 30–33.

Halliday, M. A. K., & Hassan, H. (1976). *Cohesion in English*. London: Longman.

Hodge, B. M., & Preston-Sabin, J. (Eds.). 1997) *Accommodations—Or just good teaching? Strategies for teaching college students with disabilities*. Westport, CT: Praeger Publishers.

Hoetker, J., & Brossell, G. (1989). The effects of systematic variations in essay topics on the writing performance of college freshman. *College Composition and Communication, 40*, 414–421.

Hooper, S. R., Montgomer, J., Swartz, C., Reed, M. S., Sandler, S. D., Levine, M. D. Watson, T. E., & Wasileski, T. (1994). Measurement of written language expression. In G. Reid Lyon (Ed.) *Frames of reference for the assessment of learning disabilitities: New views on measurement issues* (pp. 375–418). Baltimore, MD: Paul Brookes Publishing.

Houck, C. K., Englehard, J., & Geller, C. (1989). Self-assessment of learning and nondisabled college students: A comparative study. *Learning Disabilities Research, 5*, 61–67.

Kaufman, A. S. & Kaufman, N. L. (1986). *The Kaufman test of educational achievement*. Circle Pines, MN: AGS.

Kiewra, K. A., & Dubois, N. F. (1998). *Learning to learn: Making the transition from student to lifelong learner*. Needham Heights, MA: Allyn & Bacon.

Kirsch, I. J., Jungeblut, A., & Campbell, A. (1991). *The test of applied literacy skills for adults*. Princeton, NJ: *Educational Testing Service*.

Kolb, D. A. (1993). *Learning style inventory* (LSI–IIA). Boston: TRG Hay/McBer.

Lahey, M. (1988). *Language disorders and language development*. New York: Macmillan.

Law, J., Jr. (1998). Review of the attention deficit scales for adults. In J. C. Impara, & B. S. Plake, (Eds.), *The thirteenth mental measurements yearbook* (pp. 7–9). Lincoln, NE: Buros Institute of Mental Measurements.

Olfiesh, M. S., & McAfee, J. K., (2000). Evaluation practices for college students with learning disability. *Journal Of Learning Disabilities, 33*(1), 14–25.

Pauk, W. (1983). *How to study in college* (3rd ed). Burlington, MA: Houghton Mifflin.

Porteus, S. D. (1965). *The Porteus mazes*. San Antonio, TX: The Psychological Corporation.

Poteet, M. (1998). A review of the ERB writing assessment. In J. C. Impara & B. S. Plahe (Eds.), *The thirteenth metal measurements yearbook* (pp. 427–427). Lincoln, NE: Buros Institute of Mental Measurements.

Resnick, L. B., & Klopfer, L. E. (Eds.). (1989). *Toward the thinking curriculum: Current cognitive research*. Alexandria, VA: ASCD.

Shuy, R. (1988). Identifying dimensions of classroom language. In J. L. Green & J. O. Harkins (Eds.), *Multiple perspective analysis of classroom discourse* (Vol. 28, pp. 115–134). Norwood, NJ: Ablex.

Silliman, E., & Wilkerson, L. (1991). *Communicating for learning: Classroom observation and collaboration*. Gaithersburg, MD: Aspen.

Sparks, R. L. (2001). Foreign language learning problems of students classified as learning disabled and non-learning disabled: Is there a difference? *Topics in Language Disorders, 21*(2), 38–54.

Sternberg, R. J (1985). *Beyond I.Q.: A triarchic theory of human intelligence*. New York: Cambridge University Press.

Tattershall, S. (1997). Real world information and school concepts: Helping students make connections for understanding. In N. Nelson & B. Hoskins (Eds.), *Child-centered strategies for classroom-based intervention: An audio workshop*. San Diego, CA: Singular.

Tattershall, S., & Prendeville, J. (1995). Using familiar routines in language assessment and intervention, Tucson, AR: Communication Skill Builders. In D. Ripich & N. Creaghead (Eds.), *School Discourse*, (2nd ed.). San Diego, CA: Singular.

Taylor, (1969). *The communicative abilities of juvenile delinquents: A descriptive study*. Unpublished doctoral dissertation. Columbia, MO: University of Missouri.

Tomblin, J. B., Abbas, P. J., Records, N. L., & Brenneman, L. M. (1995). Auditory evoked responses to frequency-modulated tones in children with specific language impairment. *Journal of Speech and Hearing Research, 38*, 387–392.

Triolo, S. J., & Murphy, K. R. (1996). The attention deficit scales for adults. Bristol, PA: Bruno/Mazel, Inc.

Vellutino, F. (1979a). *Dyslexia: theory and research*. Cambridge, MA: MIT Press.

Weinstein, C. E., Palmer D. R., & Schulte, A. C. (1987). *Learning and study skills inventory*. Clearwater, FL: H & H Publishing Co.

Wiig, E. H., & Secord, W. (1992). *Test of word knowledge (TOWK)*. San Antonio, TX: The Psychological Corporation.

Wing, C., & Scholnick, E. (1981). Children's comprehension of pragmatic concepts expressed in "because," "although," "if," and "unless." *Journal of Child Language, 8*, 347–365.

Zachman, L., Barrett, M., Huisingh, R., Orman, J., & Blagden, C. (1994). *Test of problem solving*, Revised. Moline, IL: Lingui-Systems.

Index